DISABILITY AND
INCLUSIVE DEVELOPMENT

DISABILITY AND INCLUSIVE DEVELOPMENT

Editors: Tanya Barron and Penny Amerena

Design: Richard Mehl and Modi Li

Publisher: Leonard Cheshire International

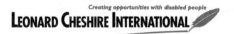

Creating opportunities with disabled people

LEONARD CHESHIRE INTERNATIONAL

Published by Leonard Cheshire International

Leonard Cheshire International
30 Millbank
London SW1P 4QD
United Kingdom

www.lcint.org.uk

© Leonard Cheshire International
February 2007

ISBN – 0-9551613-7-1
ISBN – 978-0-9551613-7-7

A catalogue record for this book is available
from the British Library.

Printed in Koramangala, Bangalore, India
by National Printing Press, www.npp.com

CONTENTS

List of abbreviations   VII

CHAPTER I: INTRODUCTION   *Tanya Barron and Penny Amerena*   I

CHAPTER 2: COMMUNITY BASED SERVICES   *Roy McConkey*   21
Section One   21
Section Two   30
Section Three   40
Section Four   58

CHAPTER 3: INCLUSIVE EDUCATION   *Susie Miles*   **69**
1. Concepts and definitions – developing a language of inclusion   69
2. History of inclusive education   72
3. Leonard Cheshire International   76
4. Key issues   77

CHAPTER 4: ECONOMIC EMPOWERMENT   *Peter Coleridge*   **III**
1. Introduction   III
2. Disabled people and poverty   112
3. International initiatives to combat poverty relevant to disabled people   116
4. Disability as a rights issue   120
5. What does empowerment mean?   124
6. The importance of economic and social context   128
7. Access to training   136
8. Access to capital   143
9. Access to jobs in the formal economy   146
10. The importance of support structures   149
11. Conclusions: pointers for action   152

CHAPTER 5: CONFLICT RECOVERY   *Maria Kett*   **155**
1. Introduction   155
2. Disability, conflict and disasters   156
3. The rights based approach to humanitarian aid and development   160
4. Conflict, disasters and community based services   166
5. Community based approaches: case study: Sierra Leone   168
6. Disability & disasters case study: Sri Lanka   176
7. Conclusions   183

NOTES ON THE CONTRIBUTORS

Roy McConkey is Professor of Learning Disability at the University of Ulster, Northern Ireland. He has worked in the field of intellectual disability for over 30 years, and this work has taken him to some 20 countries in Africa, Asia and South America.

Susie Miles is Coordinator of the Enabling Education Network (EENET) and Programme Director for the M.Ed Special and Inclusive Education at the University of Manchester.

Peter Coleridge has focused on the inclusion of disabled people in development programmes in the Middle East, Asia and Africa working for NGOs, the UN and as a freelance consultant. He is the author of the book *'Disability, Liberation and Development'*, as well as other books and articles arguing for the inclusion of disabled people in mainstream development.

Maria Kett is Research Fellow at the Leonard Cheshire Centre of Conflict Recovery (LCC), University College London.

NOTES ON THE EDITORS

Tanya Barron is the International Director of Leonard Cheshire. She is a Senior Associate Member of St. Antony's, Oxford and has worked in disability and development since 1986. She was the Chair of the UNICEF NGO Committee in Geneva for 5 years.

Penny Amerena has both a doctorate and 20 years' experience in international development. A published author, she writes for the NGO sector, particularly for development, health and disability organisations.

The editors are very grateful to Roy McConkey, Susie Miles, Peter Coleridge and Maria Kett for their contributions. We also thank Roy McConkey for his contributions to the introduction on disability models and Judith E Heumann, Jabulani Ncube and Sue Stubbs for their input. We are grateful to Sunanda Mavillipalli for providing essential input in planning the book and discussing content.

LIST OF ABBREVIATIONS

CBR	Community Based Rehabilitation
DFID	Department for International Development
DPO	Disabled People's Organisation
DPSA	Disabled People of South Africa
ERW	Explosive Remnant of War
GPDD	Global Partnership for Disability and Development
HLID	Holy Land Institute for the Deaf
IDDC	International Disability and Development Consortium
ILO	International Labour Organisation
LCC	Leonard Cheshire Centre of Conflict Recovery
LCI	Leonard Cheshire International
LPHU	Lebanese Physically Handicapped Union
MDG	Millennium Development Goal
MFI	Micro-Finance Institution
MODE	Medunsa Organisation for Disabled Entrepreneurs (SA)
NGOs	Non-Government Organisation
NUDIPU	National Union of Disabled People of Uganda
PRSP	Poverty Reduction Strategy Paper
SARS	South African Revenue Service
UNDP	United Nations Development Programme
UNESCAP	United Nations Economic & Social Commission for Asia and the Pacific
UNHCR	United Nations High Commission for Refugees
UNICEF	United Nations Children's Fund
USDC	Uganda Society for Disabled Children
VTC	Vocational Training Centre
WHO	World Health Organisation

CHAPTER I

INTRODUCTION

TANYA BARRON & PENNY AMERENA

THE PURPOSE OF THIS BOOK

The purpose of this book is to promote change, to help move policy and practice towards real inclusion and participation of disabled people.

The book also reflects frustration at the current pace of change, and the persisting absence of the meaningful participation of disabled people in development programmes. Whilst there has been some progress on involvement in policy formulation in some countries, it is still rare for disabled people to be fully involved in programme implementation. Most governments with development budgets and most NGO practitioners frame their missions and objectives in the language of social justice and inclusion. Yet few seem to notice the almost complete absence of disabled people from their agendas, priorities and programmes.

Disability and Inclusive Development is a call to action. We will only achieve inclusive development when disabled people represent themselves at all levels. Disability issues must be included in global and local development goals and processes to improve the quality of life of some of the world's most disempowered people.

WHO WILL FIND THIS BOOK USEFUL?

Disability and Inclusive Development is written for all those involved in international development as well as those working directly in the field of disability. If an overarching aim in development is to include disability issues in all development processes, then every development practitioner needs to think about, and integrate, disability issues in their work.

THIS BOOK IS FOR YOU IF YOU:

- are an international development policymaker, planner, implementer or practitioner
- work at international, national, regional or community level
- work for government, a civil society organisation or an international development organisation
- are a trainer in international development or the disability sector
- are a trainee or student in international development or the disability sector. You represent the new generation of practitioners and we hope the drawing together here of current thinking on inclusive development issues will be particularly relevant to you.

WHY INCLUSIVE DEVELOPMENT MATTERS TO US ALL

The global development community will not achieve the UN Millennium Development Goals (MDGs) by the target date of 2015. We can say this with confidence because disabled people have been left out of the equation for the MDGs relating to poverty, health and education. For example, the goal of the second MDG is to achieve universal primary education, but with 98% of disabled children excluded from school, this will be unattainable. A widely used statistic is that up to 10% of the global population is disabled and amongst them are some of the poorest and most marginalised people in the world (WHO 2006). They are excluded from the key international development targets that attract funding and drive change. It is vital to redress this omission and the invisibility of disabled people because this percentage figure represents the social exclusion of up to 600 million individuals.

Change is critical because the reality of everyday life for disabled people globally is harsh:

- 98% of children with disabilities in developing countries do not attend school[1]
- 200 million of the world's 1.2 billion poorest people surviving on a dollar a day are people with disabilities (Elwan 1999)
- 80% of disabled people in developing countries are unemployed (ILO 2003)

---

[1] Report of the Director General of UNESCO, Koichiro Matsuura, to UN Development Group 2003, www.unesco.org.

- 51% of disabled people are women and they have even less access to essential services such as health care, education and vocational rehabilitation than disabled men (Disability Awareness in Action 1996)

PUTTING INCLUSIVE DEVELOPMENT INTO PRACTICE: THE CHAPTERS

When we planned the text we aimed to inform, provoke debate and increase understanding of the range of interacting issues that operate in this complex area. More than this we wanted to provide practical ideas for improving inclusive practice in development without being prescriptive. The book contains contributions from four leading experts and commentators in the field of disability and inclusive development. The topics selected represent areas of prime importance in disability: education, economic empowerment, community services and conflict and disaster recovery.

The first three themes are probably what each reader would expect to find, but why conflict and disaster recovery? This topic is included because in an increasingly politically and naturally volatile world, war, conflict and natural disaster are becoming more common. These phenomena cause impairments and add significantly to the numbers of disabled people in the world. At the same time those individuals who have existing disabilities become even more invisible, falling through the net of relief operations. This is an area where very little has been published and we are pleased to begin to explore the implications in this book.

Our contributors have interpreted the commissioning guidelines in ways that are meaningful for them and the sectors they operate in. The result is four individual and differing perspectives that reflect the reality of each area of practice. There is, however, a common thread. For each contribution the goal is social justice. While the terminology and the way social justice might be achieved for disabled people differs for each topic, there is a united call for empowerment as a right.

This book, then, links the aspirational to the practical; it taps into what motivates development and disability workers at all levels and offers ideas on how to begin to translate guiding principles into effective action. Not everyone will agree with what they find in this book, but we hope it provokes critical reflection and renewed urgency in each reader's contribution to including disabled people in development.

COMMUNITY BASED SERVICES

Professor Roy McConkey sets out the alternative approaches of rehabilitation service provision and the issues surrounding them. We see how different approaches can co-exist in practice depending on the impairment(s) and the national or local model for working with disability. Do inclusive services always offer the best option? While he identifies strengths and weaknesses in each type of service provision, the pragmatic goal is to work with the resources that are available and strive to make them as person-centred as possible.

Despite the UN 1994 Standard Rules on the Equalization of Opportunities for Persons with Disabilities, which state that disabled people have the right to remain in their community, for some the reality is that service provision is only available in institutions that deny their rights and take them away from their families and friends. For others, service provision may be in the community, either mainstreamed through community services or through specialised services provided locally. But whether the service is delivered through an institution or in the community, disabled people often experience rehabilitation services as part of a medical model: as recipients rather than participants. So Professor McConkey's call for person-centred services recognises aspirations and capacities as well as needs, and helps practitioners extend the opportunities of rehabilitation towards empowerment. The emphasis is on fulfilling potential and enhancing quality of life while recognising resources constraints and, importantly, sensitivity to cultural factors.

INCLUSIVE EDUCATION

Susie Miles provides a valuable discussion of the key issues. Her contribution goes beyond the 'special' versus 'inclusive' education debate. In the education sector the Salamanca Statement, Education For All and MDG goals have focused attention on mainstreaming practice. It is clear that the education MDG will not be reached without increasing inclusive measures because of the current exclusion of poor and marginalised children, including disabled children, in many countries. Yet while governments' policies to include disabled children in mainstream schools have led to a quantifiable change, there has not been a corresponding evaluation of the quality of education provided. Many activists see a twin-track approach as the best way forward, where specialist services are provided alongside mainstream education, allowing mainstream teachers to be trained to offer teaching methods that meet the educational needs of all children.

The chapter explores the policies and existing activities that support access to education for children with disabilities worldwide. It also offers a range of practical factors to be considered in interpreting and implementing equitable education in different cultural contexts.

ECONOMIC EMPOWERMENT

Peter Coleridge explores the essential components of an integrated model of economic empowerment.

Disability and gender are presented as factors of heightened vulnerability, which keep people trapped in a cycle of poverty.

Whether a disabled person can earn a living or not will impact upon their sense of self-worth, fulfilment and self-determination. It is here perhaps that the interdependence between access to rehabilitation services, education and economic opportunities is most obvious. It is here also that discrimination against women may be most keenly felt, though this also exists in rehabilitation, education and conflict recovery responses.

A twin-track approach is vital in economic empowerment, where market forces will not bring about economic inclusion without government policy, programmes and legislation. Special provision of vocational training and access to micro-credit is essential to enable disabled people to start their own small businesses or enter employment.

Peter Coleridge highlights the role of advocacy, participation and the process of individual and community empowerment. In the employment sector, as in all other sectors, policies that affect disabled people are not developmental unless disabled people have been involved in the decision-making process.

CONFLICT RECOVERY

Maria Kett provides insight into the vulnerability of disabled people in fractured and disrupted societies, and examines the links between conflict and disaster, poverty and disability.

Amongst the many people affected by conflict and natural disaster, disabled people are almost invisible in relief and recovery work, and are often excluded from access to basic needs. Conflict and natural disaster phenomena have a number of impacts.

They create disability, not solely through injury or violence but also through poor health and malnutrition. They also create refugees who are amongst the most marginalised of all. People who were disabled before the conflict or disaster, along with their families, become even more neglected. These people are affected by the breakdown of basic service provision and support, and often find themselves excluded from mainstream relief and emergency operations.

Maria Kett presents Leonard Cheshire Centre of Conflict Recovery's (LCC) objectives and activities resulting from these considerations, which may provide the reader with a starting point of discussion or a template for development. In this often neglected area the chapter helps development practitioners address the process of recovery in ways which takes into account the rights and dignities of disabled people.

APPROACHES TO WORKING WITH DISABLED PEOPLE

Some contextual background and definitions are necessary to set the scene for each of the chapters that follow. First of all, what is disability? The World Health Organisation (WHO) uses the International Classification of Functioning definition:

'Disability is a generic term that includes impairments in body functions and structures, activity limitation and participation restrictions. It indicates the negative aspects of the inter-action between an individual (with a 'health condition') and his context (environmental and personal factors).' (PAHO & WHO 2006).

And impairments are *'problems in body function or structure such as deviation or loss'* (PAHO & WHO 2006). Impairments therefore refer to physical, sensory and mental problems, including illness and lack of emotional well-being.

Most definitions of disability capture the fact that bodily impairment leads to disability, which is a social construct or a result of society's reaction to the person with an impairment. Thus UNESCAP (2005) states: *'many [disabled people] are so excluded and alienated from their own society that they are no longer treated as respected 'citizens' of their own society.'*

An inclusive development approach is the global development community's response to attempt to rectify this situation. However, 'what is inclusive development?' is less easily answered. In our search for a simple form of words that captures the idea and recognises its multi-dimensionality, we asked three leaders in current thinking on disability and inclusive development to share their perspectives. They were each asked 'What is inclusive development and why is it important?' The wide-ranging contributions mirror the complexity of the topic and the challenge facing practitioners.

Judith E. Heumann, global disability strategist and advocate, Lead Consultant of the Global Partnership on Disability and Development, states:

'Put simply, the term 'inclusive development' denotes the concept that ALL stakeholders (women, children, disabled people, indigenous people, elderly etc.) have an equal right to be participants in, and beneficiaries of, the global development agenda.

For inclusive development to be effective, society as a whole must take ownership of it. Disabled people and parents, where appropriate, must be integral participants in all decision-making and implementation mechanisms. For this to happen, those mechanisms must be accessible, and disabled people and their representative organisations must also have access to the education, training, and any other capacity-building necessary for them to meaningfully contribute.'

Jabulani Ncube, an eminent disability activist from Southern Africa, proposes:

'Inclusive development ... means paying particular attention to the needs of the downtrodden and marginalised.

It means recognising that in human development processes there are asymmetries of power, access to information and capacity, which serve inexorably to drive weaker sections towards the margins. It means recognising that development means taking a stand against injustice. It requires an appreciation that social development in the context of developing countries is not a neutral subject to be discussed merely as an intellectual construct, detached from the hard terrain in which people lead their lives.'

Sue Stubbs, International Disability and Development Consortium (IDDC) Coordinator, offers the following:

'Inclusive development is a process as well as a goal...this process of development must involve and benefit all stakeholders, at every stage. Disability as an issue is both a catalyst for inclusion and a measure of its success. Inclusive development is important because it is ultimately the only approach that reflects the real potential of human society. It has many implications for practical ways of working, such as respecting different opinions, building consensus wherever possible, power-sharing, acknowledging mistakes, ensuring basic needs are met (eliminating extreme poverty), actively identifying and addressing barriers to inclusion, and most importantly, being committed to the fact of our inter-dependence, and taking collective responsibility for the realisation of the full human rights of all.'

We can draw out from these viewpoints the common thread of a demand for social justice for the marginalised and oppressed, the requirement that all stakeholders are included in development processes. There is consensus on empowerment or power-sharing. The practical issue of establishing mechanisms and resources for empowerment and participation in decision-making is highlighted. There is emphasis on the interdependent nature of human society, which underlines the need for the empowered to acknowledge responsibility to include and enable the marginalised to claim and achieve their human rights.

MODELS OF WORKING WITH DISABLED PEOPLE

How far do the models for working with disabled people match up with current thinking on the key components for inclusive development? An understanding of the broad range of international development approaches and their evolution is important. When we compare the models we notice a stark contrast between the present aim for inclusion and empowerment and how early and later models impact upon disabled people. In some ways this might seem like critically assessing development efforts against goals and standards that did not exist at the time. Yet it is highly relevant to understand and distinguish between different approaches, because many disabled people receive services and support and experience levels of participation which are influenced by historical approaches to working with disability. In fact the very word 'receive' encapsulates the problem. Practitioner attitudes towards disabled people in systems influenced by some of these approaches may be out of step with current thinking. Overwhelmingly, disabled people tend to be the 'beneficiaries': the target of what others decide they should have. They receive rather than participate. One of our aims in this book is to help practitioners question and adapt existing systems or develop new ones which address rights, needs and participation as effectively as possible within economic and human resource constraints.

THE MEDICAL MODEL

The medical model is an early approach to helping disabled people in both the developed and developing countries. Many specialist disability services around the world are based on the medical model. Few would question that what nurses, doctors and other medical specialists deliver is of tremendous importance, as they strive to address physical, sensory and mental impairments. Yet the origin and nature of the medical approach, involving diagnosis and the knock-on effect of pathologising, has produced significant problems when applied to disabled people. The medical model has therefore been criticised for focusing on the impairment and not the person, and certainly not on the society in which the disabled person lives.

In this original model it is as if the purpose of the support a disabled person receives is to enable them to adapt to society's requirements. The approach is often associated with negative ideas of:

- permanence (there is little perceived chance of meaningful change)
- dependency (the individual needs to be 'looked after')
- passivity (the disabled person is not capable of self-determination).

Disabled activists have criticised the approach because it largely ignores the social, cultural and physical environments which play a significant part in restricting life-style and level of functioning. For example in the medical model:

- disabled people's basic needs and rights such as education, employment and housing are often overlooked
- the diagnostic language categorises the individual according to conditions and symptoms and this devalues and stigmatises
- the focus is on deficit rather than talents and competencies
- the role of society in disabling people is ignored. There is no recognition that 'the individual's experience of disability is created in interaction with a physical and social world designed for non-disabled people' (Swain et al. 1993).

The medical model itself has influenced approaches to working with disabled people in contexts unrelated to medical or health institutions. For example, schools and employers may see a disabled person solely in terms of their impairment rather than viewing them as an individual with competencies and potential as well as needs. This narrow perspective is characteristic of the medical model and disability activists have fought against its widespread impact. They argue instead that four basic dimensions should be used to describe the disability experienced by each person:

- *Impairments* – physical, sensory and mental, including illnesses and emotional problems.
- *Functional limitations* – particularly those affecting day to day living such as personal care.
- *Social inclusion* – access to education, employment and community facilities, plus the barriers to inclusion they face within their communities.
- *Supports* – physical and human supports, both available and needed, which may relate closely with the factors above.

THE SOCIAL MODEL

This approach evolved initially from disabled people voicing their dissatisfaction with society's attitudes towards them. The social model sees disability as a result of the interaction between a person with an impairment and the environmental and attitudinal barriers they face. From this model's perspective society disables at least as much as the impairment.

The focus is on assessing the environment not only the impairment to identify what interventions need to be made in the environment to enable the individual to participate in society as fully as other people. For example, this might be an accommodation in the form of lifts instead of stairs or providing hearing aids. Both of these accommodations will reduce the person's experience of disability in society. Disabled activists have focused their efforts on the most meaningful determinants of social inclusion: access to education, employment and community facilities, such as transport, housing and access to public buildings.

Clearly the social model of disability aligns closely with the Declaration of Human Rights, so that assessment and treatment of the individual is related directly to addressing the barriers and providing the supports that help realise equality of opportunity.

In recent years WHO's introduction of the International Classification of Functioning, Disability and Health (2001)[2] represents a development of the social model. This

---

[2] Available from: http://www3.who.int/icf/icftemplate.cfm

framework can be used to evaluate all aspects of health and health-related components of well-being for all people, not just those related to impairments. This powerful tool therefore identifies levels of functioning in society. It does not categorise people but allows the situation of each person to be described within a range of domains and areas which affect functioning, such as health (including impairments and illnesses), environmental and personal factors. The resulting information may then be used to identify the specific support and assistance each person needs.

The social model represents a significant step forward for changing attitudes to working with disabled people. Assessment, whether in medical institutions, schools, community-based rehabilitation, employment or development projects, should now take into account the reality of the person's life and consider their lifestyle, needs and hopes for fulfilment. Assessment aims include:

- The active participation of the person in the assessment process
- Identifying a complete picture of the person with positive attributes not just deficits
- Identifying supports to remove barriers that limit access to opportunities and participation in society.

Unfortunately, despite the effort of activists to change attitudes and approaches, practice does not match guidelines in many parts of the North and South.

SEEING THE DISABLED PERSON AS AN INDIVIDUAL

A clear outcome, then, of activism and the evolution of approaches to working with disabled people is recognition of the uniqueness of the individual. This comes from acceptance of the basic fact that a particular impairment may have different impacts upon different people. Also each person lives in unique social and cultural circumstances.

This acknowledgement is influencing policy-makers and practitioners to avoid the historic tendency to group disabled people and services together. The aim now is to respond to each disabled person as an individual with unique talents, difficulties, hopes and challenges. The goal is to empower all disabled people to have choice and self-determination, where services and funding are individually matched to each person.

INDIVIDUALISED SERVICES

A central feature of individualised services is developing a person-centred plan for each individual which allows services to be matched to their needs. It moves away from bringing disabled people to services and instead aims to deliver services to the disabled person in their home or in their community. Each plan is developed actively involving the disabled person, or a representative such as a family member, as a controlling stakeholder who can voice needs, aspirations and capacities. In ideal circumstances the plan is seen as a partnership where stakeholders, including the individual, family members, relevant community workers and professional staff, jointly participate to set up the plan, deliver it, review and develop it.

This approach is therefore quite different from plans devised by professional staff under the original medical model.

PERSONALISED FUNDING

In the North many countries have state systems that offer financial allowances to individuals, following assessment of their eligibility. Increasingly, disabled people are becoming entitled to individual budgets that they control directly to pay for the support they choose. This allows each disabled person greater determination over what and whom they have in their lives to help them, instead of being allocated staff and support by a service agency.

Both the individualised service and personalised funding approaches are rare in developing countries largely because of funding implications. Yet there are examples where the ethos of self-determination can and does influence a more individualised service approach in community-based services, and where micro-financing schemes can be developed as a form of personalised funding.

THE RIGHTS-BASED APPROACH

The joint impact of changing attitudes to development and disability which urge participatory approaches, combined with the growing voices of disabled activists, has given rise to a rights-based approach to disability. Campaigners have demanded the eradication of paternalistic approaches and the recognition of each disabled person as an individual.

The social model played a key part, influencing a fundamental shift in thinking by introducing the idea of disability as a phenomenon created by society. This led to the perspective that each disabled person is not only an individual with unique needs and characteristics, but an individual who is a citizen with the same rights as any other member of society.

By 1975 the *United Nations Declaration of Rights of Disabled Persons* stated:

'Disabled persons, whatever the origin, nature or seriousness of their handicaps and disabilities, have the same fundamental rights as their fellow citizens of the same age, which implies first and foremost the right to enjoy a decent life, as normal and as full as possible.'

While this was a statement of rights it was not a call to action. Nearly twenty years later the UN in its *Standard Rules on the Equalization of Opportunities for Persons with Disabilities* (1994) set out actions that member states could implement to bring about meaningful change. In summary:

'Persons with disabilities are members of society and have the right to remain within their local communities. They should receive the support they need within the ordinary structures of education, health, employment and social services.' (Para. 26)

This was an improvement and has led to anti-discriminatory and dedicated funding legislation, particularly in resource-rich Northern countries, which partially translates aspiration into action. However the language used in these broad UN and international directives is not mandatory. National governments will not be persuaded to act when the phrasing of directives is conditional or open to wide interpretation. Directive wording such as disabled people 'should receive the support they need' or 'reasonable adjustments' will not motivate governments to act, when there are competing resource considerations and a lack of political will. The forthcoming UN Convention on the Rights and Dignities of Disabled People provides a stronger statement of actions for governments. However experience of previous human rights treaties informs us that it is difficult to persuade governments to comply on inclusive development issues.

The unresponsiveness of governments worldwide to a range of emancipatory issues is a fundamental factor in the rise of non-governmental organisations and civil society organisations to lobby and drive action. Yet change for disabled people has been slow. This raises the question why such qualifying language in UN directives has been used for the rights of disabled people when it would not have been tolerated for other marginalised groups? Perhaps part of the answer lies in the diversity of disabled people. There are many types and degrees of impairment and disabled people do not form a homogeneous group. This factor combined with the level of disempowerment and marginalisation they experience has made it more difficult for people with disabilities to mobilise as a cohesive and powerful force in advocacy, than for some other pressure groups.

The rights-based approach, nonetheless, has had a number of impacts, including:

- the rise of the disabled peoples' organisations (DPOs)
- the introduction of a mainstreaming approach.

THE RISE OF DISABLED PEOPLE'S ORGANISATIONS

Since the 1980s DPOs have both driven and been strengthened by the rights-based approach which is enshrined in the various UN Human Rights Declarations and Statements for marginalised groups generally and for disabled people specifically. Activists have followed the rights-based path for social inclusion. Advocates fought for the rights of disabled people to represent themselves and participate in decision-making rather than be represented by other organisations such as charities or non governmental organisations. This signalled a move from a social welfare (or 'a being done to') model to a rights-based approach dedicated to empowerment. This was coupled with the aim of taking responsibility in partnership, for disabled people's services and supports. Activists have challenged societies' prejudices against disabled people as 'victims', 'patients' and too 'inadequate' to perform a proactive role. Centuries of oppression and societies' embarrassment, stereo-typing and neglect has begun to be directly addressed.

DPOs exist at local, regional and national level. By linking disabled people with one another, DPOs' representative function allows them to perform important roles in:

- creating solidarity to reduce isolation and build confidence
- delivering advocacy to challenge society's attitudes and practices
- sharing information to empower members
- providing relevant services to meet members' practical needs

- providing training to raise community and service staff awareness as well as developing members' (and where relevant their families') know how and skills.

This is a complex range of roles and increasingly DPOs have organised at the regional and national level to share knowledge and skills so they can more effectively meet the needs of members at local branches.

DPOs play a vital role in empowerment yet they face common setbacks including:

- fragmentation resulting from the range of impairments and attributes the members have which may be difficult to reconcile within one organisation
- maintaining momentum because of the day to day challenges that disabled people face, and the feeling that the skills required to run an organisation may be beyond their capacity
- conflicting aims coming from members' disagreement on the purpose of the organisation which might range from advocating social justice, to improving service provision, to disagreement about special or integrated services.

Skilled leadership is required to overcome these problems and maintain focus on enabling disabled people to participate fully in society. Institutional strengthening and organisational capacity building are required at regional, national and international levels to support DPOs to negotiate and carry out their chosen roles effectively.

THE INTRODUCTION OF A MAINSTREAMING APPROACH

With growing acceptance of the idea that disability is a phenomenon created by society, disability activists have fought for the same rights, responsibilities and provision of basic needs as fellow citizens. Both campaigners and development practitioners increasingly questioned why disability policy and programmes were separated from the main development initiatives. They argued that the consequence of impairments was a disabling social exclusion and therefore disability issues should be included throughout national and international development strategies in all fields, including universal education, gender equality, maternal and child health and poverty reduction. In response, government policies for inclusion throughout the world are increasingly taking the form of 'mainstreaming'.

DFID's Disability KaR (Knowledge and Research) project offers a useful definition[3] of mainstreaming in disability:

'Mainstreaming disability into development cooperation is the process of assessing the implications for disabled people of any planned action, including legislation, policies and programmes, in all areas and at all levels. It is a strategy for making disabled people's concerns and experiences an integral dimension of the design, implementation, monitoring and evaluation of policies and programmes in all political, economic and societal spheres so that disabled people benefit equally and inequality is not perpetuated. The ultimate goal is to achieve disability equality.'

The drive for mainstreaming comes also from a recognition that mainstreaming benefits everyone in society; it is not a form of special assistance for disabled people.

Yet while development practitioners and disability organisations support the goal, many are already sceptical about the ability of the mainstreaming process to deliver meaningful inclusion in the short and medium term.

THE CURRENT CONTEXT

We have briefly outlined the development over time of the main approaches to working in the field of disability. We do not however suggest that this has been a linear progression, that global consensus now exists between policy-makers, nor that all national governments, whether in the North or South, listen and respond to disabled people's informed advice. Worldwide there is a concurrent mix of medical model, social model and rights-based approaches. These approaches may co-exist within the same country and differ between the type and severity of impairment.

Even the rights-based approach which seemed to offer so much hope has led to disillusionment among many disabled people and DPOs. The focus on advocacy is judged by some to have deflected attention, and therefore funding, away from improving the quality of life of disabled people. Advocacy is necessary but all too often disabled people have communicated their views and fought for their rights at international and national platforms, and talk has not generated social justice.

In this context of dissenting voices the rights of the individual means different things to different people. The closest point of agreement is that disabled people

---

[3] http://www.disabilitykar.net/pdfs/learn.pdf
  This definition was adapted by the Disability KaR project from UNDP's gender mainstreaming definition.

are citizens and have the right to participate fully in society. Yet while some disabled people see participation as inclusion in society, with full access to mainstream education and employment, others maintain their rights are best served by special and separate service provision, in the form, for example, of special schools and dedicated vocational training. The situation is further complicated by families who represent those disabled people who are unable to speak for themselves and who may not agree with decisions made on their behalf.

Both DPOs and development realists are coming to the conclusion that the rights-based goal of social inclusion will not be delivered by mainstreaming alone. Mainstreaming has given some disabled individuals access to schools and employment, but it has not always given equal quality of education or workplace experience.

Mainstreaming is becoming increasingly popular with governments, perhaps because it seems to both respond to the rights-based movement's demand for inclusion and to be a relatively economically attractive solution. Once this approach has been adopted it is very difficult to introduce the idea of twin-tracking where both mainstream and special provision opportunities are provided. To policy-makers twin-tracking appears inconsistent with the lobby for inclusion, and it costs more. Yet to many disabled people and development pragmatists, a twin-track approach is required to meet the rights and needs of people with disabilities, as we wait for the mainstreaming approach to translate rhetoric into reality.

THE FUTURE

Mainstreaming can be seen as a process leading to inclusion. Where the process currently fails is in its budgetary allocation (insufficient budgets are allocated to ensure that all services are truly accessible to all in the broadest sense) and in the evaluation of quality of outcomes. Do the outcomes truly represent social, economic and political inclusion for disabled people? The answer, at present, is no. Outcome measures need to more directly reflect and gauge progress against social inclusion goals for a non-homogeneous group of excluded people. For example, counting the numbers of disabled children attending a mainstream school is simply not useful if the quality of education and outcomes for the child are not measured.

LCI therefore considers that mainstreaming is currently an inadequate approach when it is applied in isolation. IDDC (2004) proposes that *'The full human rights of disabled persons will not be realised without a twin-track approach to promoting Inclusive Development*', and identifies two key components in the twin-track approach to inclusion:

- Removing existing institutional, environmental and attitudinal barriers to social inclusion, as well as creating new systems that are non-discriminatory and barrier-free. The mainstreaming approach of 'disability proofing' development programmes is a necessary tool, but achieving social inclusion goes far beyond these sorts of measures, aiming to bring about attitudinal and behavioural changes in society.

- Empowering the individual and the organisations that represent them. Capacity building is an essential component of social inclusion so that individuals have access to basic information, skills and support (including relevant services) to improve the quality of their lives. This is the component that is most often overlooked in the current trend for mainstreaming policies: inclusion must have meaningful impact on the quality of life of the individual.

In the current development context a combined mainstreaming and twin-tracking approach offers a way to achieve social inclusion and deliver the rights of the disabled person to participate fully in society. It attends to the rights, aspirations and capacities of the individual while not overlooking the need for supports and services.

How and when will this happen? Without the political mobilisation of disabled people, change is likely to be slow. The reality of the world is that economic power generally equals political power in the North and the South. Those that hold economic power rarely take action to contribute to the empowerment of marginalised people unless there is an incentive. This places a disparate, disempowered group like disabled people at an enormous disadvantage. Change will require two essential driving factors:

- the mobilisation of disabled people: the momentum of disabled people focused on finding their voice, articulating their rights and needs and truly participating in decision-making processes.

- the mobilisation of resources: progress on social inclusion will only be achieved hand in hand with appropriate levels of funding in the development process. We should shine the spotlight on examples of weak political will for social justice, where there is no evidence of budgetary or financial provision to implement inclusion.

There are several ways that disabled people and DPOs can mobilise to empower themselves:

- by forming lobbying alliances with other marginalised groups to achieve power in numbers and fight for legislative change
- by working with non-disabled allies, not to be represented by them, but to access support such as capacity-building within DPOs
- by achieving an attitudinal change towards themselves which will influence other people.

This last point may seem contentious. It may appear to put the onus unfairly on disabled people and in fact there is diverging opinion on the issue. But we are persuaded by, for example, Peter Coleridge's study of disability in *Disability, Liberation and Development,*

'The truth is the oppressor is not likely to change behaviour unless the oppressed person makes the first move ... If [disabled people] refuse to see themselves as victims, if they claim their own dignity, see themselves as positive and able to contribute, they will be seen as positive and able to contribute. This is not at all the same as saying that disabled people should be quiet, stop complaining, and settle for some kind of half life. Absolutely not ... In the words of Rachel Hurst of Disabled Peoples' International: "Social change initially comes from us, from disabled people. It has to."'

CONCLUSION

Our aim is to generate action. The exclusion of disabled people from social, economic, political and community life is perpetuated by ignorance and poverty, and exacerbated by conflict. Without change at all levels disabled people will continue to be largely excluded from the development process. Without their active participation in decision-making, development efforts will not be relevant. This disempowerment leads to loss for both the individual and the community where each would benefit from unlocking the potential of disabled people.

Whether you agree or disagree with the content of this book we hope it motivates you to evaluate the sector you work in and stimulates action to increase the rate of progress towards inclusive development.

REFERENCES

Coleridge, P., 1993. *Disability, Liberation and Development.* Oxford: Oxfam.

Disability Awareness in Action, 1996. Disabled Women, Resource Kit No 6. London: Disability Awareness in Action. Available from: http://www.independentliving.org/docs2/daakit61.html#anchorcontents

Elwan, A., 1999. *Poverty and Disability: a background paper for the World Development Report.* Washington: World Bank.

IDDC, 2004. *Inclusive Development and the UN Convention.* *IDDC reflection paper,* p3. Available from: http://www.un.org/esa/socdev/enable/rights/ahc3iddc.pdf

ILO, 2003. *Time for Equality in Work.* Geneva: ILO

Pan American Health Organisation & WHO, 2006. Disability: Prevention and Rehabilitation in the Context of the Right to the Enjoyment of the Highest Attainable Standard of Health and Other Related Rights. In: *138th Session of the Executive Committee, Washington D.C., 19-23 June 2006. Provisional agenda item 4.7.* Washington DC: PAHO & WHO, p.4. Available from: http://www.paho.org/English/GOV/CE/ce138-15-e.pdf

Swain, J., Finkelstein, V., French, S. and Oliver, M., 1993. *Disabling Barriers – Enabling Environments.* Milton Keynes: Sage Publications and Open University.

UNESCAP, 2005. The strategic approaches to disability development. *Regional Workshop on Comprehensive National Plan of Action on Disability, 19-21 October 2005.* Bangkok, BMF. Available from: http://www.worldenable.net/bmf2005/basicdoc3.htm

WHO, 2006. *Disability and rehabilitation WHO action plan 2006-2011.* Geneva: WHO. Available from: http://www.who.int/disabilities/publications/dar_action_plan_2006to2011.pdf

CHAPTER 2

COMMUNITY BASED SERVICES

ROY McCONKEY

SECTION I

LIVES WORTH LIVING

Disability is all too often represented in terms of sadness and despair, of helplessness and hopelessness. Indeed many appeals to charitable giving are based around such descriptions.

Yet this is not the reality of many families and persons living with a disability. They too experience joy and fulfilment, happiness and contentment. They do not view their impairments as a personal tragedy but rather they come to see them as part of who they are (Swain and French 2000). For them, life certainly is worth living.

> The non-tragic view of disability… is about disability as a positive personal and collective identity, and disabled people leading fulfilled and satisfying lives. Swain & French (2000)

In this section we explore in more detail what makes for a fulfilling life. Armed with this information we can look critically at the quality of the lives of people with a disability (whether they are living with families, in residential settings or in their own accommodation), and see how their lives could be improved.

At the outset we must stress two important truths that link back to issues discussed in the Introduction:

- Human lives and lifestyles are culturally determined. Hence aspects of people's lives that are especially valued in one culture may not be valued in another culture;

- Humans vary in what is important to them. Hence even within the same culture some people will place greater value on certain aspects of life than will other people.

People with disabilities are not immune from either of these truths. As we stressed in the Introduction, the key is to focus on the individual we are supporting and to plan with them how best we can assist them, taking full account also of the culture of which they are a part.

DIMENSIONS OF LIVING

In more affluent countries, the concept of 'quality of life' has received much attention. The aspiration towards a better life is ever-present and on certain indicators undoubtedly there have been marked improvements in people's living standards, with better housing, greater choice of food and near full employment. But some would argue that these material benefits do not necessarily translate into a better quality of life.

Recent research and debate has identified eight core dimensions that contribute to a person's quality of life (see Table 1). We need to remember that:

- These dimensions are largely distinct although they do impact on each other. This means that meeting a person's need on one dimension, such as their material well-being, does not produce gains on other dimensions;

- The dimensions are not arranged in any particular order because the salience of each dimension will change from person-to-person. Emotional well-being may be a critical dimension for one person whereas another is more concerned with rights;

- People's priorities will also change over time and with different circumstances. Their physical well-being may be central for a time but as these needs are met, issues around self-determination may come to the fore;

- These dimensions apply equally to people supporting persons with disabilities, most obviously to family members, but also to paid staff working in services. If we can improve their lives, we could reasonably expect people with disabilities to also benefit.

TABLE I: QUALITY OF LIFE INDICATORS (Shalock and Keith 2000)

Dimension	Content	Indicators
Emotional well-being	Safety	Freedom from stress
	Spirituality	Self-concept
	Happiness	Contentment
Inter-personal relations	Intimacy	Interactions
	Affection	Friendships
	Family	Supports
Material well-being	Ownership	Employment
	Financial Security	Possessions
	Food	Socio-economic status
		Shelter
Personal development	Education	Personal competence
	Skills	Purposeful activity
	Fulfilment	Advancement
Physical well-being	Health	Health care
	Nutrition	Health insurance
	Recreation	Leisure
	Mobility	Activities of daily living
Self-determination	Autonomy	Personal control
	Choices	Self-direction
	Decisions	Personal goals and values
Social inclusion	Acceptance	Community activities
	Status	Roles
	Supports	Volunteer activities
	Work	Residential environment
Rights	Privacy	Due process
	Voting	Ownership
	Access	Civic responsibility

This framework or some version of it can help us in a number of ways.

Firstly, it can be used to review with the person how they view their life at present. The indicators noted in Table 1 are some of the tangible ways the person can identify the good and 'not-so-good' aspects of their lives. We need to focus on what the person and/or the family sees as important (sometimes called their subjective appraisal) and beware of imposing our priorities on them. For example, people may be content to remain living in shanty accommodation because they value the supports they get from their neighbours although by objective standards their accommodation is very much sub-standard.

Secondly, it defines the range of supports that people with disabilities may require in order to live more fulfilling lives. For example, services may focus on improving people's material well-being and meeting their health needs. These may be necessary and vital supports but by themselves they are unlikely to provide the full solution. Indeed there may even be the danger that services that focus only on certain aspects of a person's life, may actually worsen other aspects of their life, such as their social inclusion and self-determination. Hence we need to place our specific endeavours within a broader perspective and either widen our service remit or else form alliances with others who can address other dimensions of people's lives.

Thirdly, this framework can help us to define the aims and aspirations of services we offer to people with disabilities while also providing a way of evaluating the quality of the service we offer them. To take the latter first, various means have been developed for reviewing with people who use a service, the different ways in which it has helped them and those aspects where further help is required. This might be done by undertaking a review with each person individually or by creating an overall review of the service to identify common strengths and weaknesses across most people who use it (McConkey 1996). In both instances, a quality of life framework provides a holistic basis for these reviews.

Similarly this framework can help us decide what the particular priorities for the service that is provided are, realising that it is very difficult to meet all the diverse needs of people with disabilities. These can then be made explicit within the service's statement of aims so that people coming to the service will have a clear understanding of what it can do to assist them.

Fourthly, and perhaps most significantly, a quality of life framework provides a common language for everyone involved with the person and the family. In particular it provides agencies which have limited involvement with disability a means of relating to the needs of people with disabilities in terms they can understand and without the medico-social jargon that has built up in the disability sector.

Likewise it encourages disability services to look beyond the narrow confines of impairment and appreciate the broader impact that disability can have on people's lives and the need to address these issues if possible within their services.

Finally, the quality of life framework applies to everyone and may be particularly helpful in assessing the needs of families looking after a disabled relative (Brown and Brown 2003). This is a theme we shall take up more fully in the next section.

QUALITY OF SERVICES

Although special services are commonly found for people with disabilities in more affluent countries this is not the case in poorer countries. Indeed internationally increased attention is being paid to equipping mainstream services to better support people with disabilities. However the quality of these services in relation to people with disabilities, but also for all the people who use them, may need to be improved. This is equally true for specialist services. In some instances they offer a very poor quality of service.

The following three broad approaches are used in assessing the quality of services.

1. Service Standards

One approach to improving quality has been to focus on attributes of the service that is provided. Very often these have taken the form of 'quality standards' that the service is expected to achieve. These may be set internally by the provider organisation or in more affluent countries be laid down by governments who wish to protect the users of services from poor care and treatment (Koornneef 2001).

The standards often reflect what is considered good, important or of value to the people requiring the service. They may cover the standard of the buildings, the food provided, staffing arrangements, activities provided and so on. Ideally the standards will have been developed in partnership with people in the service, their families and experienced staff and they should take account of cultural norms. For example in many affluent countries, a standard for residential accommodation is that each person should have their own bedroom. This may not be appropriate in other cultures.

The standards set by government also have to be attuned to the available resources within the society. This is a careful balancing act. If the standards are set too high, then services that are adequate will be deemed to fail but equally if the standards are set too low, unacceptable services will not improve.

EXAMPLE OF NATIONAL CARE STANDARDS IN SCOTLAND FOR CARE HOMES FOR PEOPLE WITH INTELLECTUAL DISABILITIES

Standard 12: Your social, cultural and religious beliefs or faith are respected. You are able to live your life in keeping with these beliefs.

1. You are given the opportunity and support you may need to practise your beliefs, including keeping in touch with your faith community.
2. Staff make sure they are properly informed about the implications of your social, cultural and religious belief or faith for you and other people living in the care home.
3. Your holy days and festivals, birthdays and personal anniversaries are recognised and ways found to make sure you can mark and celebrate these as you choose.
4. The social events, entertainment and activities provided by the care home will be organised so that you can join in if you want to.

Different standards have been developed for various forms of services. Thus, the standards used in a residential home are different from those developed for early intervention services or vocational training centres. Nonetheless there are often a common set of standards that apply in all settings.

Adopting a core set of standards is also a means for organisations to express what they hold in common. This can apply to branches of the same organisation or when autonomous organisations want to affiliate to a broader body.

2. Performance Indicators

Performance indicators are another approach that can be used to assess services. These focus more on the management procedures that are thought to result in good quality services, for example financial stability, low staff turn-over, number of people seen by the service and user engagement. Internationally the best known is probably ISO 9000[4] although in Europe various other systems are also available, such as EFQM[5].

These systems are designed to assess public and private organisations and not specifically those for people with disabilities. In response to criticisms, more attention is now paid to the outcomes for consumers of services although the main focus remains on how managers comply with stated procedures.

3. Personal Outcomes

This approach identifies a number of outcomes that people using the service could expect to receive. These may derive from past research, the aspirations of present consumers or those set by the service providers. They are a statement of the specific 'goals' for the service as opposed to the broader aims or vision for it. For example, the Council for Leadership and Quality in the United States has produced 25 personal outcomes that services for people with an intellectual disability are expected to produce for the people they serve (Gardner and Carran 2005).

EXAMPLES OF PERSONAL OUTCOMES

- People live in integrated environments.
- People participate in the life of the community.
- People interact with other members of the community.
- People perform different social roles.
- People have friends.
- People are respected.

Assessing the Quality of Services

Devising a set of service standards or performance indicators is only a beginning. More crucial is how the service is assessed against these standards. This can be done in different ways including the following options.

---

[4] http://www.iso.ch

[5] European Foundation for Quality Management (1999)

- Feedback from consumers: often the onus is left with individual people to complain if the service is not meeting the standard they expect from it. Procedures are laid down for doing this either verbally or in writing, and the quality standard will require service-managers to respond to the complainant. This approach may become confrontational but it does pinpoint specific instances of bad practice.

- Sometimes individuals are reluctant to complain in case they are victimised. This can be overcome through access to independent advocates or by encouraging the formation of advocacy groups of people using the service.

- Better still is to inculcate in staff an attitude of continual checking with the people using the service as to how they feel about it.

- Managerial reviews: the people who manage the service (whether in a paid capacity or as volunteers), have a responsibility to ensure that the standards are being met in the day-to-day running of the service. Ideally their checks will be based on first-hand observations although they may also rely on reports from staff in the service and from the people using it. A high reliance is placed on the managers to perform this function and some may be reluctant to do it. Also if the manager is the reason for the poor service, how will this be identified?

- Service reviews: all the people involved with the service – managers, staff and service users – come together to review how the service is performing and identify ways of improving it. This could be done on an annual basis. Outside facilitators may be recruited to assist with this. This approach often gets used when a service is in 'crisis' but it has value for all services (McConkey 1996).

- Inspections: outside inspectors, such as individuals appointed by governments, visit the services to check that standards are being met. This approach has long been used in schools and in businesses, for example, when auditors come to inspect the financial accounts. Inspectors should be knowledgeable about services with experience of working in them. Although they may be there to find fault, a more important role is to guide the service or to how it could improve.

Of course it is possible and indeed it is desirable to use a combination of methods for evaluating the quality of services on offer to people with disabilities. But there have been some concerns that quality services do not result in improved quality of lives for people with disabilities.

One of the main reasons is that the focus of service evaluation is often on the setting in which the service takes place or on the activities that the services offers. From the provider's perspective these may be important, but if the standards do not result in better outcomes for the person using the service, how much do they actually count? This brings us back to the quality of life frameworks with their key indicators and the individual approaches in services described earlier.

A lot of what can be counted doesn't count. A lot of what counts can't be counted.
Albert Einstein

CONCLUSIONS TO SECTION ONE

- Enhancing the quality of life of people with disabilities is a daunting prospect particularly in societies in which poverty and deprivation are rife. Nonetheless remarkable progress has been made all over the world in doing this for at least a few people. These examples can inspire and guide us in making this happen for more people, in more countries, more of the time.

- There is growing awareness of the need to regularly review the standard or quality of services provided to individuals, whether they are government funded or provided through volunteer effort. This will check that the needs of people are being met and help identify better ways of making this happen.

- In some respects the key resource for improving people's quality of life is not money, important as that is, but rather social networks and relationships with other people who are prepared to give their time and talents to support people in need. That is the focus of the next section.

SECTION 2

SUPPORTING FAMILIES

In all countries of the world, families provide the bulk of support for children with disabilities and in many instances this continues into the adult years as well. Thus to support people with disabilities in the community means supporting their families. They are the main resource found in every community throughout the world.

Often it is mothers who shoulder most of the responsibility with the eldest sister doing more than her fair share. Grandmothers and aunts may step in as well. However their caring role has to be done alongside many other demands on their time: household chores, income generation and caring for aging parents (Gartner et al. 1991).

Indeed society has found it impossible to replicate the level of love and devotion that families bestow on their relatives with disabilities. In affluent countries, children's homes have closed in favour of finding alternative families such as foster carers and adoptive parents. But in many poorer countries, there is often no alternative to care by relatives.

Thus a basic priority underlying all our service provision in community settings must be to boost the resources of families to care for their relatives. In this section we shall explore ways of doing this.

Families also provide us with an example of the type of relationships we need to nurture in support of people with disabilities. This includes relationships with volunteers and with paid staff as well as with other people who have a disability.

AN IRREPLACEABLE RESOURCE

In many countries, families provide the only care that people with disabilities receive. This scenario is unlikely to change in the foreseeable future.

* Families do their best often with meagre resources but many lack the knowledge and skills to most effectively help their relative. They need information.

* Families may struggle to cope with the day-to-day demands of caring for their relative which could be made easier if they had access to more appropriate aids, appliances and support. They need practical assistance.

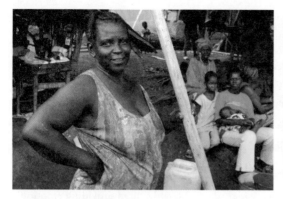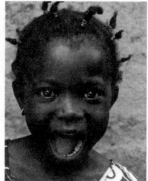

Photos: Jenny Matthews / Leonard Cheshire

- Families can become stressed and exhausted from the demands placed on them. They need emotional support.

It is a tribute to the resilience of the human spirit that so many families do manage to cope under the most trying of circumstances. However it is at a cost to both themselves and their relatives in that the quality of their lives is often so poor (Balasundaram 1995).

Removing the person from the family may appear an attractive solution and in some instances may become a necessary one if the disabled relative is being neglected or abused. However when resources are scarce it is often not a practical solution and in many instances it is not a desirable one.

- The fulltime care of a person outside of the family is much more expensive and it can be a life-long commitment. Hence fewer people will be able to be helped if monies are limited.

- When people leave their family, especially in childhood, the family often loses touch with them and can be reluctant to bring them home again. Likewise the person with disabilities loses familiarity with the family or their home community and may prefer to stay in the place they know.

- If given a choice, families often prefer to continue caring for their disabled relative if they can get some assistance locally rather than sending the person away. The same is true for people with disabilities, probably even more so.

Hence the primary response of all disability services must be to support families, to work to retain people within families and to maintain family links when people move away from their families.

Internationally, several approaches have proved successful in supporting families. We shall consider each in turn:

Family Support Workers: in Western countries, one of the success stories of modern disability services has been the advent of home visiting schemes in which a trained worker regularly visits the family to advise on ways of promoting the child's development. They are known by many different terms: home visitors, home therapists, CBR worker, but in this paper the term 'family support worker' is used for this role.

- With experience their role has widened considerably, often providing emotional support to mothers, giving advice on other family matters and acting as an advocate for the family. Among the best known schemes are those based on a model originating in Portage, USA but now used in many other countries (Meisels and Shonkoff 2000).

- Around the same time, the World Health Organisation started to promote the concept of Community-Based Rehabilitation (CBR) as a means of helping people with disabilities in the developing world (United Nations 1994b). Here too, a trained worker, who may be paid or unpaid, visits the person with a disability at home to show the families what they can do to help their disabled relative and to offer the family support and encouragement. We will explore further this form of service option in Section Four.

- Although the evidence remains equivocal on the impact such home-based programmes have on the development of the person with disabilities, there is widespread agreement that they are valued highly by families. James Gallagher (1992) attributed this to "a new spirit of optimism and encouragement within the family", replacing the despair and feelings of hopelessness that usually flow from disability.

- Family support workers are not a new concept. The extended family or 'clan' has often provided an advisor or confidante to new mothers with whom they can discuss their concerns. The home visiting idea builds on this tradition by introducing the family to a person who has particular expertise or interest in the disability. However cultures vary in their tolerance of an 'outsider' becoming involved in family issues and services must be sensitive to this when recruiting staff to act as family support workers (Jaffer and Jaffer 1990).

- *Recruiting family support workers:* family support workers can be recruited from at least three different sources and, around the world, projects invariably use some combination of these. Firstly, existing personnel are re-deployed to act as family support workers. Teachers, therapists and health workers have adopted this new style of working rather than seeing people solely in hospital clinics or disability centres.

- Secondly, family support workers are paid employees having been recruited and trained specifically for this role. Although the original idea was to recruit people from the community, more recently an increasing number of people with disabilities or parents of children with disabilities have successfully been employed as family support workers (McGlade and Acquino 1995). This strategy not only gives much needed employment opportunities but these individuals come with personal insights and motivation which can make them more effective and acceptable to families.

- Volunteer workers form a third option. Some community services use family members as their primary workers whereas other community schemes have successfully recruited teachers and health workers, among others, to act as voluntary supporters for families. This is best exemplified in Brian O'Toole's (1995) work in Guyana.

However, it is the qualities that the home visitor brings to the job rather than the background from which they come that ultimately appears to contribute more to their effectiveness. In particular, it is important that:

- They have an empathy with the culture of the family. Families are then more accepting and trusting of them;

- They respond practically to the family's needs. Parents and the disabled relative should experience some immediate benefits from having a home visitor;

- They try to involve all family members. Grandparents, siblings and cousins can all be recruited to assist with the child with a disability;

- They empower families to be decision-makers. They should share information and expertise freely with families so that they are empowered to make decisions and solve their problems.

Although the options for finding effective family support workers are available in most communities around the world, a great deal of effort needs to be expended on recruiting suitable individuals, while recognising the inevitable turn-over which occurs with poorly paid or volunteer workers.

This approach of providing personal supports to families and people with disabilities is now widely accepted in developed countries as a means of giving carers extra help at home or short breaks from caring as well as enabling people with disabilities to live independently in what has become known as 'supported living'.

Parent Associations: bringing parents together in local, regional or international associations has been another success story. Usually the groups have formed around specific impairments such as cerebral palsy or hearing loss. They may also vary in size and sophistication. Many were begun by parents with help from professionals.

Most parent associations pre-date the formation of DPOs and they continue to have a key role in advocating for children. However there can be tensions between parent associations and DPOs as they may have different priorities, concerns and dynamics among their memberships.

Parent associations commonly fulfil three main functions similar to DPOs: providing parents with solidarity, information and advocacy (Skogmo 1995).

- Solidarity: the heart-ache that comes from feeling isolated with a problem can be assuaged by meeting others who have been through or who are going through similar experiences. Indeed the literature is full of examples showing that parents and families often feel isolated and unsupported even in well developed communities. Membership provides the emotional support for mothers when it is not forthcoming from other family members. They can also help to create a sense of pride in having a child with disability. Solidarity appears to be best fostered at a local level; hence national parent associations need to develop a network of branches.

- Information: parents bemoan the lack of information that is available to them even when they have access to a range of professionals (Chen and Simeonsson 1994). Often the need is for information that is tailored to their present needs and concerns and presented to parents in readily accessible ways. In Lesotho, southern Africa, the leaders of nine parent group branches linked to the national parent associations, identified six main needs for their parents (McConkey and Mphole 2000) (see box).

Parent associations often produce newsletters for their members; most organise meetings, conferences and training events with invited speakers; some have telephone help-lines and others employ 'parent advisers' or development workers to provide information and training for their members. These appear invaluable for many families which are often eager to know how they can provide better care, support and importantly, interventions for their relative.

- Advocacy: national associations have a vital role to play in speaking up for the rights of people with disabilities. Parent associations often organise events to profile issues of concern and gain the interest of media such as radio and newspapers (McConkey et al. 2000). Delegations from the association may also meet government officials to press their case. Likewise, the national association may support individual members as they confront local issues, such as school enrolment or the example of police refusing to prosecute a rapist of a woman with intellectual disabilities. The advocacy role is likely to be more effective if alliances are made with other organisations who share a common interest, most notably organisations of people with disabilities. In many countries there is now some form of national disability council that brings together all the disability organisations.

Parent associations can take on other important roles such as fund-raising and provision of specific services to families, but the three core functions should remain the bed-rock of their purpose.

THE MAIN NEEDS OF PARENT GROUPS IN LESOTHO

- Knowing how to assess, teach, train and handle their child
- Ways of raising parental awareness and of mobilising parents
- Rights of people with disability
- Disability issues generally
- Working alongside professionals, report writing for committee members
- Making teaching aids and equipment

A key role for professionals working in communities is to help nurture parent associations if there are none available in the area (McConkey and Alant 2005).

Families need a break from their caring role and equally the person with disabilities needs to experience a world beyond the family. Hence the importance of enrolling children in any available pre-school facility, nursery school or ordinary school. Other options have included the development of some form of day provision for children, including a crèche, nursery, school, or day centre. Adults also benefit from daytime training centres and workshops.

These services meet the needs of parents in various ways:

- Their relative is looked after for a period of time which gives the family carer the opportunity to do other things, notably earn some income. This can be crucial in enabling families to survive. Some disability services deliberately develop income generating schemes for parents as part of their services. South Africa provides the example of a community group that opened a centre for children with multiple disabilities who were not allowed access to the local schools. In an adjoining room they had a sewing shop for mothers to make school uniforms which were sold in the local community. Similarly, in the Philippines a revolving loan scheme was made available to mothers who had children with severe visual impairments so that they could earn an income at home (Campos 1995).

- The family carers meet other families facing similar challenges. These informal contacts offer some of the benefits of parent associations noted earlier or they might be formalised into a parent association linked with the service. Opportunities are also created for carers to learn how other families are coping and to benefit from their experiences.

- The family carers have access to staff in the service from whom they can get advice, information and support. These opportunities can be maximised if service staff also visit families at home or they set aside time to regularly meet with the family carers and to review how things are going at home as well as in the centre.

However the services should also benefit the individual with the disability, for example in the following ways:

- Meeting other people: although obvious and often taken for granted, this is a core function of any form of out-of-home activity. Meeting other people encourages communication, provides role models and develops friendships. A range of activities are more fun when done in groups rather than alone.

- Learning new skills: the rationale for most schools and centres is not just to look after the person, but to actively help them to acquire new skills. This should reduce the disabling effects of their disability and equip them to become more self-reliant. A priority is for people to become mobile, to have a means of communication and to look after their personal care needs, self-feeding, toileting and washing. They can also be taught basic house-hold chores such as simple cooking and washing clothes, so that they make a positive contribution to the family and free up other members for other activities.

- Receiving specific treatments: in centres, people can get specific therapy or treatments as required by the nature of their impairments which can be done more cost-effectively than at home. For example, a physiotherapist can assess, treat and review a number of children on one visit to a centre and show the staff and the family carers how they might continue the therapy until their next visit. Other specialists may be employed in the centre, to provide ongoing treatments for the children and adults although this option is mostly confined to more affluent countries. Indeed even then, some would question the efficacy of this approach if the therapy is not maintained by family at home.

An ongoing debate surrounds the extent to which these support services need to be solely for people with disabilities or whether the same or better outcomes can be achieved through the use of services provided for everyone in the community. We shall examine this issue in the next section.

What is not in dispute is the need for services that support families while assisting the family carers. Indeed even when the child or adult is living away from the family in a boarding school or residential centre, family contacts must be maintained.

This is harder to achieve because of the distances involved and the expenses of travel, but the same methods noted earlier apply here too: home visits by staff, regular contact with staff by telephone or review meetings, and invitations to events when families can meet one another. And when children and adults have no contact with their natural families, volunteer substitutes may be found in the adjoining community such as 'foster aunts and uncles'.

The goal is simply stated: to enable every person with a disability to have the experience of being a member of a family. This very fact opens the door to so many opportunities which professionalised services struggle to provide.

BUILDING SOCIAL NETWORKS

The family is also the basis for the development of social networks in the wider community. Everyone benefits from having social contacts outside of the family but these are even more crucial for people when they have no contact with their own families.

A support network is made up of people who socially interact. This broad definition is useful as it reminds us that we all belong to many different networks and we enter and leave various networks in the course of any day. It is through these networks that acquaintances are built, friendships develop and more intimate relationships can evolve. Hence social networks are vital for creating social lives. Arguably people with disabilities have an even greater need than non-disabled persons to have a network of social supporters. Even so many are denied the opportunity of loving relationships, marriage and having children, largely because of negative attitudes within society.

Social networks vary in terms of size, intimacy and longevity, often reflecting the personal aspirations of the person at the heart of them. But for most people with disabilities, their networks tend to be smaller, more dense (the same people feature) and with more unreciprocated relationships. Many are overly reliant on one or two people (usually a family member or staff person) for companionship and in fact there are some who are friendless.

This had led some disability services to try and develop a 'circle of support' or a 'circle of friends' around the person with a disability (Neville et al. 2000). There is no prescription for the form and format these take as they will be guided very much by the wishes and needs of the person with disability as identified in their person-centred plan. That said there are some common strands in such circles:

• they might include family members, siblings, cousins, aunts and uncles; neighbours and acquaintances; co-workers for people in work settings; members of clubs, churches and so on who know the person. The size of the circle does not matter; a few interested people can make a start. The circle does *not* have professional workers as members although they can have a key role as facilitators in creating the circle;

- it is likely that the depth of friendship will vary across the members of the circle. Some may be prepared to be intimately involved; others will continue as acquaintances but they will be better informed than previously;

- the circle might meet from time-to-time to explore with the person and each other the contributions they are making to each other's lives. Members of the circle may help with transport, others can seek out work opportunities and some may act as social companions. In many ways this is the old idea of the mutually supportive tribe recreated for societies where the bonds of kinship have weakened.

In developed countries the idea of a circle of support has found expression in different ways. For example a housing provider, which supports people with disabilities to live independently, builds up mutually supportive networks among the tenants living within a geographical area as well as linking them into the communities where they live (Simons 1998). They are encouraged to help each other with a range of tasks or chores rather than relying on paid staff to do so.

Community is a place of belonging where people find their identity (Vanier 1991)

CONCLUSIONS TO SECTION TWO

- The quality of life of most people is heavily determined by their social relationships. In the face of great adversity, the companionship of others can be an invaluable solace. But as Vanier (1991) reminds us, our relationships with families and other people in a community give us a sense of emotional security and of belonging. This is how we create a sense of who we are.

- If we are to be true to our vision of everyone being people first, and disabled second, then we need to find ways of affirming everyone's personhood through the time-honoured ways of membership of families and communities. If however these bonds are broken or never nurtured, then the risk is that the only identity people attain is that of being disabled.

SECTION 3

MODELS OF SERVICE PROVISION

Throughout the previous three sections we have illustrated how the needs of people with disabilities can be met in different ways and the key role that families and communities can play in doing this alongside the contribution of disability services specialising in this area.

In this section we examine the variety of models that now exist for helping people with disabilities. In essence they range along a continuum from highly specialised services at one end to services that are available to everyone in the community, and through which the needs of people with disabilities are addressed. However there is a considerable degree of overlap now emerging between these models.

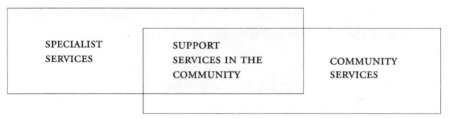

Figure 1

In past decades, the priority was to develop specialised services, otherwise people with disabilities were ignored and neglected. However in recent years the focus has shifted towards community services mainly because of a realisation that specialist service models cannot cope with the sheer numbers of people requiring help, as well as recognition that it is both possible to meet people's needs in ordinary community settings and indeed, it is also their right.

Initially a specific model of Community-Based Rehabilitation (CBR) Services was proposed as an alternative to the dominant model of Institution-Based Rehabilitation (IBR) (Helander 1993). Experience has shown, however, that community based approaches are more effective when they are tailored to existing resources within specific communities and allied with the needs of the people with disabilities in the local area, rather than trying to replicate a particular model of service delivery or one based around a particular ideology (Mitchell 1999a).

We made clear in the previous section, families still provide most of the care and support to their relative with a disability. This is especially so in poorer countries, but it is still a reality in most affluent nations. Hence the primary function of many services set up to assist people with disabilities, whether they are specialist or community-based, is for them to act in support of individuals and their family members.

The three main service options (see Figure 1) will now be examined in turn.

I. SPECIALIST SERVICES

The origin of many specialist services was in response to people with disabilities who were orphaned or whose family were unable or unwilling to care for them. Unable to fend for themselves many died, were destitute or survived through begging. A common response throughout the world was the provision of places of 'asylum' where the children and adults had at least their basic needs met for protection and shelter (Felce 1996). However another reason for such provision was that of protecting society from individuals who could pose a danger to others, such as people with Hansen's disease or with a mental illness, or those who provoked feelings of shame and disgrace such as children with an intellectual disability.

Although many hospitals, homes or institutions were started by charitable organisations, these became the bedrock of early provision by governments. Indeed many people in society will still view such places as the archetype of services for people with disabilities. This may be because they see such individuals as helpless and in need of specialist care, or perhaps such centres serve to reinforce these images of people with disabilities.

As more funding has become available, the form and function of many institutional services has evolved in the following ways.

- People living in such centres are offered education, training and therapy to overcome their disabilities. Special boarding schools for children with disabilities are a good example of this changed ethos, but adult centres have also embraced it. This has enabled people to obtain work outside of the centres and even to move out into other living arrangements.

- The centres have created opportunities for people to attend on a day basis to benefit from their services, particularly people who live with their families.

Alternatively organisations have opened special day centres to meet the needs of this group. These include special schools, day centres, vocational training centres and sheltered workshops.

- Some centres have refocused their efforts into the provision of short-term treatment. People are offered places for a limited period of time during which they will receive treatments, therapy and training that will enable them to function better in their home community. Family carers may also attend for training as well. An example would be rehabilitation centres for people with acquired disabilities. However the idea has been extended in different ways, for example to prepare people for living independently, to offer training for certain careers and to obtain educational qualifications. This model promotes a through-put of people so that more people have the opportunity to access a service. Otherwise special services often fill up, so that no more admissions are possible, even for people whose needs may be greater than those already in the service.

- To these three models of specialist services we can add the original one of the provision of care, because throughout the world, there are still many services that continue to offer only this. However there is widespread agreement this model of service is insufficient and that it denies disabled people their right to an ordinary life.

"If the stay of a disabled person in a specialised establishment is indispensable, the environment and living conditions therein shall be as close as possible to those of the normal life of a person of his or her age". UN Rights of Disabled Persons, 1975

While the form and function of specialist services have changed in recent years, two things have remained constant:

- Firstly, the services are exclusively for people with disabilities and often strict admission criteria are laid down to reinforce this. Moreover the services tend to concentrate on particular groupings often defined in terms of impairments such as services for people with physical disabilities, or for hearing difficulties, or those with intellectual disabilities. Indeed people with more than one type of impairment may then experience some difficulty in getting the services they require.

- Secondly, the people who work in the service often receive special training to equip them for the work or else they acquire their expertise through working on-the-job. A wide range of professions may be involved in services within developed countries, typically nurses, therapists, doctors, psychologists and social workers. They too may specialise in certain disabilities and some may have taken specialised training for these posts. The 'professionalisation' of disability services has helped to create the impression that specialist expertise is always required to support people who have a disability.

However as we see later, specialist services have evolved yet further as they work in partnership with community agencies. Nonetheless these two features still distinguish their contribution.

THE STRENGTHS AND WEAKNESSES OF SPECIALIST SERVICES

The strengths of specialist provision can be summarised as follows:

- they allow expertise to be developed in assessing and supporting people with particular disabilities;
- they provide a visible point of reference for people to seek help and a tangible reminder to the community of the need for specialised assistance;
- a sense of camaraderie and a common identity can be nurtured among people who use the service;
- funding for the service is more likely to be assured on a continuing basis; especially of longer-established services;
- people accepted into the service have some reassurance that the service will continue even though staff may come and go.

Equally the shortcomings associated with specialist provision are becoming more apparent. These include:

- a limitation on the number of people who can use the service;
- specialist services are usually located in cities and towns which mean they are often not accessible to people living in rural areas;
- the high costs associated with establishing new services;
- poorer people may not be able to afford the costs if financial contributions are required by the service;
- the expertise around disability is not shared with others who may be better placed to prevent disabilities or ameliorate their impact in people's lives;
- they perpetuate the exclusion and segregation of disabled people from community life.

These shortcomings have prompted interest in finding alternative ways of providing services. The most radical approach has questioned the basic assumptions around the necessity for specialist provision and promoted the idea that the needs of people with disabilities could be met within ordinary settings using the same services, such as health and education, which are available to everyone.

2. COMMUNITY SERVICES

Community services focus primarily on people living with family carers or those living in their own accommodation, which they may share with a few other persons. In any one locality the number of persons with marked disabilities (excluding the elderly) is probably no greater than 5 per 100. Hence there are not large numbers of people who would overwhelm existing services, which is a fear expressed by some. However the types and severity of their disabilities can be varied so they may challenge services in different ways.

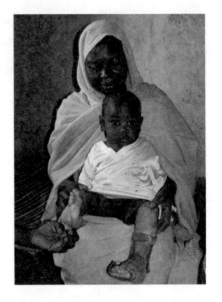

Inclusive services: the inclusion or 'mainstreaming option' as it has been termed, depends on equipping existing community personnel, such as teachers and health staff, and services such as clinics and schools, to meet the bulk of needs of people with disabilities.

This option is furthest developed within education and it aims to ensure equal access to the same opportunities that are available to non-disabled persons while retaining people within their communities rather than segregating them from the rest of society albeit with the best of intentions, namely to meet their special needs (Miles 2005).

Mainstreaming can feature in all aspects of life, notably in meeting the social and leisure needs of persons with disabilities, their need for productive work and opportunities for housing. The UN Standard Rules on the Equalization of

Opportunities for Persons with Disabilities spells out how this can be done (United Nations 1994).

Of course specialists in supporting people with disabilities are still required. They certainly have a key role to play in training staff in community services. They may also act as consultants for staff if they encounter particular problems and they could even be appointed to the mainstream agency to provide ongoing support and assistance to the staff. Equally the best specialist advisors are often disabled people themselves. They and their relatives can guide and advise others.

STRENGTHS AND WEAKNESSES OF THE MAINSTREAM MODEL

In many ways the mainstream community model reflects the opposite strengths and weaknesses of the specialist approach.

The strengths are:

* people remain within their families and communities;
* universal coverage is possible including in rural areas;
* the extra costs are considerably less;
* the service is more attuned to the particular cultural and social needs of people with disabilities;
* negative attitudes and stereotypes in the community are challenged.

The weaknesses are:
* the needs of people with disabilities are ignored due to other work pressures;
* staff in mainstream services are reluctant to take on extra responsibilities when they already feel over-worked;
* the expertise is lacking to give people with the disabilities the help they require; especially those with more severe conditions;
* it is harder to bring people together into parent associations or DPOs.

If 'pure' specialist services and 'pure' community services have contrasting strengths and weaknesses, then the solution is obvious: take the best of both! This is happening the world-over, though from differing starting points. We shall next look at how specialist services are reaching out in communities and then at how community services have developed more specialist provision for people with disabilities.

3. SUPPORT SERVICES IN THE COMMUNITY

Specialist services have evolved into community-based services in different ways. These attempt to retain some of the strengths of specialist provision while responding to the unmet needs of people in many countries through the judicious deployment of scarce specialist resources. These options can be inter-related and one may grow out of another.

SPECIALIST OPTIONS

CLINIC OUTREACH

SPECIAL UNITS

THERAPY AIDES

SEEDING NEW SERVICES

Clinic outreach

One common approach is for specialists such as therapists to base their assessment and treatment clinics in community facilities rather than specialist settings, using local health centres or school classrooms or community halls instead of hospital clinics.

Indeed a small team of specialists may visit different locations on a rota basis, say once a month. However an important corollary of this approach is to have a cadre of local people working with the team, such as community health workers, so that they can encourage families to attend the clinics as well as to provide some follow-up support to them (see below).

This approach is good at giving specialists an insight into the family and community life of the person with the disability and for building personal relationships with community personnel. However, this approach does not provide for ongoing support of families unless the team returns regularly to the locality.

Special units attached to mainstream facilities

This option has been favoured by some educationalists attempting to meet the needs of children with disabilities in ordinary schools when there is reluctance to include children in the classes. For example, a classroom for these individuals is established in the local school and ideally a teacher with particular expertise is appointed to teach the pupils.

Similarly disability resource units linked to district hospitals have been provided with specialists on hand to offer assessments and treatments rather than having families travelling long distances to hospitals and clinics in major cities.

These units can serve a number of additional functions, notably the provision of local training courses for families and community personnel. However a recurring problem is the recruitment of suitably qualified staff and retaining them in their posts especially in more rural areas. These positions do not have very high status within professions.

Recruitment and training of 'therapy aides' to work in community settings

Another option has been to create a new category of professional worker who works under the supervision of specialists and who has been trained specifically to deal with more 'routine work', and for this to be done across a variety of disciplines. For example they will receive basic physiotherapy and occupational therapy as well as communication training.

These community-based staff are recruited from local communities and based there fulltime, so they are able to build up trusted relationships with families and community personnel. However they may refer people to the specialists with whom they are linked as well as receiving supervision and monitoring from them. However in under-resourced services the latter dimensions may be overlooked.

The development of suitable training courses for this grade of worker has not been easy to resolve as it does not fall under the remit of any existing specialism. Nonetheless, Zimbabwe provides an example of working in this way. Likewise some health systems are reluctant to create a new grade of worker.

Seeding new services

Another role that specialist centres can play is to help 'seed' new facilities or services in their locality or in another district. The experience and expertise of staff can be made available to others wishing to develop a similar service. In this instance the specialist service acts mainly as a consultant to the new group, providing them with advice and training as needed and perhaps even seconding staff for time-limited periods. However the new service remains autonomous although they may enter into some form of federal relationship with the founding organisation.

Leonard Cheshire used this strategy to good effect when establishing homes in other countries[6]. Likewise the Indian Institute for Cerebral Palsy based in Kolkatta, India has helped to seed a number of partner agencies throughout West Bengal[7].

This strategy not only ensures that greater numbers of people can be helped, but it increases the number of organisations promoting their cause at a local level.

GUIDELINES FOR SHIFTING
FROM SPECIALIST TO COMMUNITY SERVICE

In many ways it is safer and easier for specialist services to continue doing what they have always done. It requires vision, energy and a certain amount of bravery to review present practices and develop new approaches. But all services benefit from a reassessment of their purpose and practices. Pretending that there is no need for change is a sure route to ultimate extinction.

Here are some of the ways specialist services have refocused their services:

- consulting regularly with the people using the service to better understand their needs;
- considering the needs of people with disabilities who receive little or no help, perhaps they are living in the vicinity of the service;
- identifying what the service does well and find ways of sharing these approaches with others who can make use of this expertise, such as family carers and interested staff in community services;
- identifying partners who can assist you in better realising your goals;
- developing an action plan and reviewing progress regularly to learn from your successes as well as failures.

The reluctance of rehabilitation professionals to take on these new roles and to change long-established ways of working has been a major impediment to developing community-based services (Kendall et al. 2000). Likewise the dearth of suitable training experiences for managers of these new styles of disability services is a major handicap facing existing disability services in the developing world.

---

[6] www.leonard-chesire.org

[7] www.iicpindia.com

EQUIPPING COMMUNITY SERVICES FOR SPECIALIST WORK

A contrasting approach is to start with a local community and find ways of overcoming the shortcomings of relying on existing mainstream service provision that were described earlier. This is preferred by many people with disabilities and their families and is more conducive to inclusion.

Three strategies have been used to help communities develop greater expertise in assisting people with disabilities. Each requires access to specialists but in these instances they are either employed by or report to community-managed organisations rather than being employed as part of specialist service systems. Often their main contribution is in training personnel working in community services.

COMMUNITY SUPPORTS:

COMMUNITY-MANAGED SERVICES

HOME-BASED SERVICES

SELF-HELP GROUPS

Community-managed services

When there are no suitable existing services within communities to assist people with disabilities, an option is then to create a new service but to make it one that is managed and owned by local personnel rather than specialists. Thus the trend in community-based rehabilitation is to ensure that people with disabilities, family members and interested local people are supported to form their own organisation rather than having specialists designing and implementing these services for them (Turmusani et al. 2001).

In Guyana, for example, local CBR committees established multi-functional resource centres where young people had training in vocational and social skills as part of a range of activities, as well as providing home supports for family carers (O'Toole 1995) (see below) .

This approach requires an emphasis on capacity building among local people and a willingness on their part to take on the responsibilities involved in running an organisation, especially when paid staff are employed. There is the danger too of a lack of continuity in service provision when leaders relinquish their posts with no one available to continue their work.

There is the risk also that such services may segregate recipients from mainstream services unless close links are maintained.

Home-based services

Another approach is to create a community service that is not based in a building but rather is centred around the person within his or her family and local community. The main service-provider in the model is a local person who has received extra training in order to fulfil the role of offering information, practical guidance and emotional support to the person with the disability and his or her family. This concept lay at the heart of what the World Health Organisation termed 'Community Based Rehabilitation' (CBR) (Helander 1993).

These workers, sometimes paid and other times volunteers, are known by various terms – CBR workers, family support workers, local supervisors – but essentially their tasks are similar. They advise and guide the person or family on coping with the disability. This may mean informing families about the help that is available in the locality, such as hospital and clinic check-ups. They may recommend equipment or aids to assist the person or demonstrate exercises or learning activities, which the family can use at home to help the person acquire new skills. They could seek out opportunities within local communities for people to get jobs or further training. However a key role is to empower the family in overcoming its own problems and mobilising the different family members in doing this.

As we noted earlier, by visiting the family regularly, for example every two or three weeks, the home visitor can build a trusted relationship with the carers, usually the person's mother or grandmother. Their role may then extend into one of counselling carers, listening to their concerns and advising on marital difficulties, financial problems and hurtful reactions of family members or neighbours. The fact that they come from the same culture as the beneficiaries tends to make them all the more acceptable.

Some CBR services set out to employ people with disabilities or parents of children with disabilities for these roles, or experienced mothers from deprived communities to assist other families in these communities. Family support workers can relate much more readily than specialists to families and can be more easily contacted by them.

The role can be demanding and the effectiveness of home visitors will depend not only on their personal qualities but also on the training they receive. This can range from short courses lasting around four to six weeks to year-long training courses. A list of the key topics required by family support workers is given in the box (Thorburn and Marfo 1990). A range of supporting manuals and guidebooks have been developed to assist them and these are a valuable resource for any service (see Appendix 1).

A major role of specialist staff is the training and supervision of family support workers. Preferably this should be done by personnel who have direct experience of providing home-based supports rather than clinic-based personnel.

This model has much to commend it and appears to have been most successful internationally in providing early intervention to children with disabilities (Meisels and Shonkoff 2000).

SUGGESTED TOPICS IN THE TRAINING OF COMMUNITY SUPPORT WORKERS

- service philosophies and goals
- exploration of one's own attitudes to disability
- skills in screening and identifying different disabilities
- effects of different disabilities on child development
- referrals to hospitals, schools etc.
- listening to and counselling families
- community attitudes to disability and factors in change
- assessing resources available in the local community
- beliefs about, and stages in, child development
- socialisation and communication
- encouraging self-care skills
- play activities and playthings
- aids and adaptations
- physical exercises
- coping with epilepsy
- behaviour management
- designing an individual programme plan
- observation and recording
- teaching skills

(Thorburn and Marfo 1990)

Its shortcomings are also apparent:

- people with disabilities may not get the specialist help they require unless linkages are formed with the requisite specialist services;

- the recruitment and retention of appropriate personnel can be difficult as there are no recognised salary scales and career structures for these workers (Lorenzo 1994);

- it has proved difficult to establish these services effectively on a regional or national basis although certain countries appear to have achieved this based around government structures (Mitchell 1999b);

- these services are very much driven by personalities and the services often collapse when they move on (Turmusani et al. 2002).

Self-help Groups

A final type of community service is when groups of people with a disability or the parents of children with a disability come together to help themselves. This is a time-honoured means in human society for like-minded people to express their faith, share their leisure time or promote their cause and protect their rights as in the case of trade unions. In this sense, self-help groups are very much a community endeavour.

They may take the form of an association to promote awareness and advocacy for persons with disabilities as we have discussed in the Introduction. Or the group members may provide a mutual service for one another, such as a crèche or preschool facility that enables mothers to attend to other chores while their child is looked after. Or the focus may be on income generation with the group working together as a cooperative to produce and market goods and then sharing the profits.

Although examples of such groups exist in most countries, their impact is often limited to small-scale initiatives that come from the drive and enthusiasm of a few individuals. It can be hard to kindle these qualities in societies marked by poverty and deprivation (Kendall et al. 2000).

An option then is for the self-help group to affiliate to a wider organisation that will provide support and resources, such as political parties, trade unions or religious bodies. As the group grows stronger it can become more autonomous.

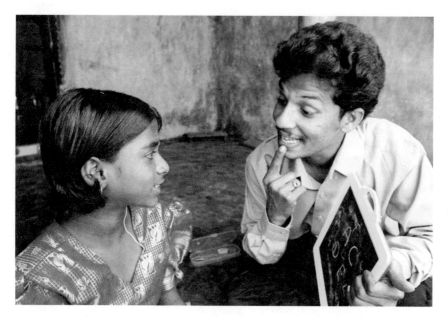

GUIDELINES FOR MAKING COMMUNITY SERVICES MORE SPECIALIST

The key requirement is having people within communities working to promote the cause of people with disabilities. Change must come from within. It is unlikely to succeed if it originates from outsiders and even less so from non-nationals. The main promoters have often been relatives of people with disabilities, often mothers, or interested professionals such as health workers or teachers who had a particular interest in this issue.

The strategies they have used include:

- identifying the resources that already exist within communities (sometimes called a situational analysis), telling them of your ambitions and listening to their concerns;
- identifying the influential people who might open doors, such as local politicians, religious leaders or village elders;
- finding out if the needs of people with disabilities are shared with other groups and forming alliances with them to argue your case, such as women's groups, unemployed youth;
- providing awareness-raising events around the issue of disabilities and training opportunities for staff in community services.

KEY POINTS ON SERVICE MODELS

A variety of service models have been examined in this section. Many of these overlap and interlink and, of course, one agency may well use a number of different models within the services they provide. Equally, different models are available to meet local circumstances and needs.

Two main conclusions stand out:

- all services ultimately depend more on the people who work in services (whether in a paid or voluntary capacity), than they do on buildings and equipment. Hence the essential task of any service is to recruit and retain people with a commitment to helping people with a disability;

- the expertise involved in helping people overcome their disabilities needs to widely shared rather than becoming the prerogative of any professional group or discipline. There is, therefore, a need for training opportunities to be available across communities and specialist services.

Viewed in this way, every community throughout the world has the potential to provide a better service to people with disabilities. This provides grounds for optimism provided these insights are communicated widely throughout all societies – to politicians, civil servants and disability specialists as well as to disbled activists, family carers and community service staff. The problems of disability can be transformed into the potentials of disability.

COMMON OBSTACLES AND CHALLENGES

Although a wealth of experience has been generated around how best to meet the needs of people with disabilities and their families, there are, however, some issues that to date have proved very difficult to overcome. Some stem from broader societal arrangements but others result from the way disability services have evolved. Of course these play off one another, but for clarity they have been grouped into two categories: disability and societal issues.

The obstacles are not insurmountable but they do present formidable challenges both locally and nationally. At present they reduce the likelihood of providing for a better life for all the people who need it, most of whom live in less affluent countries. Creative solutions no doubt will be found to them in time and a starting point is to describe the nature of the challenge.

Charitable image

A charitable image of disability is still promoted internationally to raise funds for services. This perpetuates the notion of helpless people who depend on other's largesse for survival and blunts arguments around empowerment and rights. Are there other ways of obtaining funds for services that can stress people's ability to help themselves and their role as contributors to society and communities? Certainly these are the messages that need to be conveyed more in the media and by word-of-mouth as well as in the style of services provided to people.

Competition and fragmentation

Disability initiatives are bedevilled by the fragmentation of effort across different disability groups. Some represent the interests of particular client groups, physically disabled, visually impaired, or hearing impaired to name but three. Organisations for people with disabilities (led mostly by so-called able-bodied people) may be in conflict with organisations of disabled persons (that is run by people with disabilities). Non-governmental agencies may be critical of government-run services and vice versa. Consequently much time and energy can be devoted to promoting the cause of a sectional interest rather than finding common issues on which to work jointly.

Professional protectionism

An industry has grown up around people with disabilities especially in more affluent countries in which paid workers can dictate who gets a service, where it is delivered and by whom. There may be strict demarcations about what each professional may or may not do. Such protectionism reduces the spread of knowledge and gives the impression that non-professionals have little to contribute. It may also lead policy-makers to invest in service structures that are not cost-effective.

Professionals need to be 'on-tap' not 'on-top' for people with disabilities. David Werner.

Finding service staff

The bulk of support for people with disabilities is provided by women in poorly paid jobs. This is just as true in the developed world as in developing countries. Moreover as affluent countries reach full employment, they find it increasingly hard to recruit and retain staff. They may then come to rely on recruiting immigrants from other countries, who may have limited awareness of local cultures and languages. The root cause may be lack of money, but it is not the full story. The work can be made more satisfying through the provision of training, support and career opportunities. However we have much to learn about putting this into practice.

Complexity of disability

People with more severe or multiple disabilities are surviving longer thanks to advances in medical science. Yet families and communities struggle to adequately meet their needs even in affluent nations. Fulltime professional care is very expensive and means that less money is then available for other people. There is no easy solution to this dilemma. Early identification and intervention may lessen the disabling effects of certain impairments. Likewise the prevention of illness such as cerebral malaria would help too, and would generate more tolerant attitudes within society. Ultimately though the needs of these individuals will need to feature in all service plans.

Residential provision

The most costly form of service is providing a home for people with disabilities if they cannot live on their own or with their families. These costs can be life-long and may increase as individuals age and they become more dependent on others. If these services are cash-limited then the quality of care provided can be very poor. More cost-effective ways have included recruiting alternative families to provide care and boosting people's ability to live independently with less support.

Leadership in services

Services for people with disabilities, where they exist, face many changes arising from our altered understanding of their needs. Likewise if no services exist at present, then there is the opportunity to develop a service that could be quite different from those established elsewhere. The challenge is to find people who can lead these changed services. People with vision are needed but more importantly who can communicate that vision to others and inspire them to join in (Zollers et al. 1999). People with determination are needed to overcome the many obstacles that invariably arise. People with expertise and wisdom are needed who can develop the skills of others. Not surprisingly such talent is in short supply and more worryingly many of our existing training opportunities in the field of disability do not engender these qualities in the people they train.

Lack of priority

People with disabilities are not a priority concern of governments and international agencies. Their value is often assessed in terms of their economic contribution to society when they may be viewed as a drain on resources rather than having the capacity to contribute. This weakens efforts at promoting the advocacy and empowerment of disabled persons. The increased emphasis on their rights is a useful counterpoint, as are examples of the socio-economic contributions that people with disabilities can make to their communities if given the opportunity to do so. Fundamentally though, these negative views stem from old notions of disability that may take generations to change. Equally political and financial systems need to be better informed about disability issues.

HIV/AIDS

In certain countries the impact of HIV/AIDS has had major implications for people with disabilities. Some will have lost their mothers and their care has passed on to other family members, often aging grandparents, but others have been abandoned and forced to fend for themselves by begging. Women may have become infected through rape in the mistaken belief that sexual intercourse with virgins is a cure for AIDS. The needs of persons with disabilities must feature in AIDS campaigns and programmes to alleviate the impact of this disease.

Recruiting volunteers

Internationally much voluntary effort has created and sustained many different services for people with disabilities. Their contribution has proved invaluable and could never be replaced by a professionalised workforce. Yet experience worldwide suggests that it is becoming more difficult to recruit people to serve on management committees, to act as family support workers, to assist in schools, centres or residential homes and so on. There is no immediate solution but this issue does deserve greater attention than it has received to date.

Government structures

The responsibility for people with disabilities may be shared across different government departments both at the level of local as well as central government. This can lead to confusion about who is responsible for the provision of services with little or no coherent planning across sectors. Disability should not be the responsibility of just one department, rather all departments have a contribution to make: education, health, social services, women's affairs, community development and employment. Possible solutions include more inter-departmental working and having a national plan that clarifies the various responsibilities of all the departments and government agencies. However these issues may have low priority for many governments.

CONCLUSIONS TO SECTION THREE

- Disability must be considered within a cultural and community context. This can ensure that many more people with a disability will receive some form of support and assistance, and yet there is the danger that their particular needs are not considered a priority unless a specialist service is provided. We will live with this tension for many years to come.

- Nonetheless creative solutions have been found to age-old problems thanks to the vision and vigour of disabled and non-disabled activists around the world. This will continue especially if the needs of persons with disabilities and of families become more closely aligned with those of other marginalised groups around the world.

The greatest discovery of my generation is that human beings can alter their lives by altering their attitudes of mind. William James

SECTION 4

CHALLENGES TO DISABILITY SERVICES

In this final section, most of the key issues identified in this discussion paper are summarised in the form of eight performance indicators that challenge any disability service to review its thinking and practice.

These are written in the form of questions followed by examples of explicit actions which the service might take to demonstrate its commitment to the stated aim. These actions are intended to be observable and hence open to scrutiny. However the actual form each action might take could be debated and challenged.

Not all the indicators will be appropriate to all services, but perhaps the responsibility should be placed on a particular service to justify their exemption.

One danger of this approach is that existing services may be left with a sense of failure. This is not intended. Many services were conceived and developed at a time when our thinking and practices regarding disability were different from current thinking. Hence these indicators point to ways in which services can further evolve to meet new expectations and different circumstances.

Equally there are many other facets of service delivery that continue to be required and existing services may well excel in this. As these are generally acknowledged, they are not listed here as a challenge facing future services.

EIGHT CHALLENGES AND PERFORMANCE INDICATORS

1. Empowerment of people with disabilities

To what extent is the service committed to empowering people with disabilities?

Possible indicators of this commitment are:

- the formation of active User Committees within services;
- the encouragement of people to join DPOs in the locality;
- the membership of people with disabilities on service management committees;
- recruiting people with disabilities to the workforce;
- the development of person-centred plans and reviews;
- moving to more individualised funding arrangements with people controlling the way money is spent on them

2. Social Inclusion of people with disabilities

To what extent is the service committed to the social inclusion of people with disabilities?

Possible indicators of this commitment are:

- the number of children supported in mainstream crèches, preschools, schools and colleges;
- the number of adults in mainstream vocational training centres or work placements;

- providing training and support to personnel in community services;
- encouraging membership in community societies by people with disabilities;
- forming partnerships with community groups.

3. Engagement with families

To what extent does the service support family carers and encourage family involvement in services?

Possible indicators of this commitment would include

- the formation of information and resource centres for families;
- encouraging the development of parent associations;
- providing early assessment and intervention services for families through home-based approaches or clinic outreach services;
- re-establishing or maintaining contacts with relatives of people in residential homes;
- replacing boarding schools with community-based support projects;
- providing home support services to people living with their families rather than bringing people into residential homes.

4. Forming alliances

How committed is the service to working in partnerships with other like-minded groups in the community, especially with DPOs?

Possible indicators of this commitment would be:

- knowing personally the key people in all the agencies within the local area;
- working together with community agencies to identify the major issues that need to be addressed;
- formulating an agreed, inter-agency action plan for taking forward these issues;
- assisting other agencies in tangible ways to further their work and being willing to invite them to do the same for the service.

5. Community needs

How committed is the service to helping in some way all persons with a disability in their neighbourhood?

Possible indicators would include:

- finding out the numbers and characteristics of people with disabilities in a designated area;
- determining their priority needs;
- liaising with community leaders and government officials about how they could be helped;
- mobilising self-help groups among the families and persons identified;
- providing on a small-scale basis some new community services with a view to having them taken over by another agency;
- developing proposals for new community services and seeking funds for them.

6. Community awareness

How committed is the service to making local communities aware of changed perceptions of disability and to lobbying politicians and government officials for action?

Possible indicators would include:

- regular use of the media to publicise disability issues and project more positive images other than charitable images;
- engaging in disability awareness training in schools and with community groups such as employers;
- offering school-leavers 'job tasters' and work experience placements;
- developing befriending and volunteering schemes;
- recruiting new members to the management committee and retiring those people who have been uninvolved;
- inviting politicians and officials to significant events in the service;
- writing letters to newspapers and participating in telephone phone-ins in radio programmes;
- linking with political parties on policy development;
- lobbying for a place on government committees.

7. Staff training

How committed is the service to a well-trained workforce imbued with the core values of respect for the dignity of all persons and equality of opportunity?

Possible indictors would include:

- having clear job descriptions for all posts (both paid and unpaid) within the service;
- offering formal induction training for all new workers that stresses the values underpinning the service;
- providing training for staff in key aspects of care as determined by the needs of disabled people and involving people with disabilities as trainers;
- offering new staff a mentor to whom they can turn for guidance and advice;
- undertaking staff supervision so that they receive feedback on their work;
- striving to develop career enhancements for staff;
- employing more disabled people on an equal basis.

8. Widening access to services

How committed is the service to making itself available to as many people as possible and to encouraging service users to become less dependent on the service and even to move on?

Recognising that the demand for services is often greater than the places available, services need to take some of the following actions to achieve this goal:

- the statement of service goals should include a commitment to help people become less dependent on the service and to 'move on';
- all new persons joining the service should be made aware that their place is time-limited and that their need for the service will be reviewed;
- in residential settings people are prepared for living independently through taking responsibility for running the home;
- people are encouraged and assisted to find paid employment so that they can become more financially independent;
- people are helped to find suitable living accommodation with other families, with friends or as a married couple;
- assistance is given to disabled people and their families to initiate and manage their own support services.

CONCLUSIONS TO SECTION FOUR

- Although disability has occurred in every generation of recorded history, we are among the first generation to see potential beyond the evident limitations that arise from biological impairments or the aftermath of illnesses and accidents.

- In many ways, the feasibility of this endeavour has been amply demonstrated as increasing numbers of people with disabilities have obtained educational qualifications, found paid employment, married and started their families.

- Equally there are many unresolved challenges, not least the potential of realising similar accomplishments in less affluent societies.

- However the directions for the journey have been identified and we can travel in hope.

APPENDIX I: SUGGESTED FURTHER READING

Alant, E. & Lloyd, L.L., 2005. *Augmentative and alternative communication and severe disabilities: Beyond Poverty.* London: Whurr Publishers.

Brown, R.I., Baine, D. and Neufeldt, A.H. (eds), 1996. *Beyond basic care: Special education and community rehabilitation in low income countries.* North Park, Ont: Captus Press.

Coleridge, P., 1993. *Disability, Liberation and Development.* Oxford: Oxfam.

Gartner, A., Lipsky, D.K., & Turnbull, A., 1991. *Supporting Families with a Child with a Disability: An International Outlook.* Baltimore: Paul Brookes Publishing.

Helander, E., Mendis, P., Nelson, G. and Goerdt, A., 1989. *Training Disabled Persons in the Community.* Geneva: World Health Organisation.

Helander, E., 1993. *Prejudice and Dignity: An Introduction to Community Based Rehabilitation.* Geneva: UNDP.

McConkey, R., 2001. *Understanding and responding to children's needs in inclusive classrooms: A guide for teachers.* Paris, UNESCO.

O'Toole, B. and McConkey, R., 1995. *Innovations in Developing Countries for People with Disabilities*. Chorley: Lisieux Hall Publications (Available on-line at www.eenet.org.uk)

Stone, E., 1999. *Disability and Development: learning from action and research on disability in the majority world*. Leeds: Disability Press.

Thorburn, M. and Marfo, K., 1990. *Practical approaches to childhood disability in developing countries: Insights from experience and research*. St John's: Memorial University of Newfoundland.

Turnbull, A.P., Brown, I., Turnbull, H.R., Braddock, L., 2004. *Families and People with Mental Retardation and Quality of Life: International Perspectives*. Washington, DC: American Association on Mental Retardation.

Werner, D., 1987. *Disabled Village Children*. Palo Alto, CA: Hesperian Foundation.

Zinkin, P. & McConachie, H. (eds.), 1995. *Disabled Children and Developing Countries*. London: Mackeith Press.

REFERENCES

Albrecht, G.L. (ed), 2005. *Encyclopedia of Disability*. Thousand Oaks, California: Sage Publications.

American Association on Mental Retardation, 2004. *Supports Intensity Scale*. Washington: AAMR.

Balasundaram, P., 1995. Fostering parental involvement. In B.J. O'Toole & R. McConkey (eds.) *Innovations in Developing Countries for People with Disabilities*. Chorley, Lancs.: Lisieux Hall Publications.

Bickenbach, J.E, Chatterji, S., Badley, E.M. and Ustun, T.B., 1999. Models of disablement, universalism and the international classification of impairments, disabilities and handicaps. *Social Science & Medicine*, 48, 1173-1187.

Brown, I. and Brown, R.I., 2003. *Quality of Life and Disability: An Approach for Community Practitioners. Chapter 8: Quality of life of families*. London: Jessica Kingsley Publishers.

Campos, M., 1995. Developing livelihoods. In B.J. O'Toole & R. McConkey (eds.) *Innovations in Developing Countries for People with Disabilities*. Chorley, Lancs.: Lisieux Hall Publications.

Chen, J. and Simeonsson, R.J., 1994. Child disability and family needs in the People's Republic of China. *International Journal of Rehabilitation Research*, 17, 25-38.

Chenoweth, L. and Stehlik, D., 2004. Implications of social capital for the inclusion of people with disabilities and families in community life. *International Journal of Inclusive Education*, 8, 59-72.

Coleridge, P., 2005. *Economic Empowerment: A Discussion Paper.* London: Leonard Cheshire International.

Donoghue, C., 2003. Challenging the authority of the medical definition of disability: An analysis of the resistance to the social constructionist paradigm. *Disability and Society,* 18, 199-208.

Durkan, M., 2002. The epidemiology of developmental disabilities in low-income countries. *Mental Retardation and Developmental Disabilities Research Reviews*, 8, 206-211.

Elwan, A., 1999. Poverty and disability: A survey of the literature. *World Development Report.* Washington DC: World Bank

European Foundation for Quality Management, 1999. *The EFQM Excellence Model. Public and Voluntary Sector,* Brussels: EFQM.

Felce, D., 1996. Changing residential services: from institutions to ordinary living, in P. Mittler & V. Sinason (eds.) *Changing Policy and Practice for People with Learning Disabilities.* London: Cassell.

Fujiura, G.T., 2004. Disability epidemiology in the developing world. *Journal of Intellectual Disability Research*, 48, 283.

Gallagher, J.J., 1992 'Longitudinal interventions: Virtues and limitations'. In Thompson, T. & Hupp, S.C. (Eds.) *Saving Children at Risk: Poverty and Disabilities.* Newbury Park, CA: Sage Publications

Gardner, J.F. and Carran, D.T., 2005. Attainment of personal outcomes by persons with developmental disabilities. *Mental Retardation,* 43, 157-174.

Gartner, A., Lipsky, D.K. and Turnbull, A., 1991. *Supporting Families with a Child with a Disability: An International Outlook.* Baltimore: Paul Brookes Publishing.

Handy, C., 2000. *Understanding Voluntary Organisations: How to make them function effectively.* London: Penguin Business.

Helander, E., 1993. *Prejudice and Dignity: An introduction to community-based rehabilitation.* New York: UNDP.

Jaffer, R. and Jaffer, R., 1990. The WHO-CBR approach: Programme or Ideology – Some reflections from the CBR experience in the Punjab, Pakistan. In Thorburn, M.J. & Marfo, K. (Eds.) *Practical approaches to Childhood Disability in Developing Countries: Insights from Experience and Research.* St John's: Memorial University of Newfoundland.

Kendall, E., Buys, N. and Larner, J., 2000. Community-based service-delivery in rehabilitation: the promise and the paradox. *Disability and Rehabilitation,* 22, 435-445.

Kisanji, J., 1995. Attiudes and beliefs about disability in Tanzania. In B.J. O'Toole & R. McConkey (eds.) *Innovations in Developing Countries for People with Disabilities.* Chorley, Lancs.: Lisieux Hall Publications.

Koornneef, E., 2001. *Development of Standard Models: a review of international and national models of processes for developing standards.* Dublin: National Disability Authority.

Lorenzo, T. 1994., The identification of continuing education needs for community rehabilitation workers in a rural health district in the Republic of South Africa, *International Journal of Rehabilitation Research,* 17, 241-250.

McConkey, R., 1996. *Innovations in evaluating services for people with intellectual disabilities.* Chorley, Lancs: Lisieux Hall Publications.

McConkey, R. and Alant, E., 2005. Promoting leadership and advocacy. In E. Alant & L.L.Lloyd (eds) *Augmentative and alternative communication and severe disabilities; Beyond poverty.* London: Whurr Publishers.

McConkey, R., Mariga, L., Braadland, N. & Mphole, P., 2000. Parents as trainers about disability in low income countries. *International Journal of Disability, Development and Education,* 47, 309-317.

McConkey, R. & Mphole, P., 2000. Training needs in developing countries: Experiences from Lesotho. *International Journal of Rehabilitation Research*, 23, 119-123.

McGlade, B. and Acquino, R., 1995. Mothers of disabled children as CBR workers. In B.J. O'Toole, B. & R. McConkey (eds.) *Innovations in Developing Countries for People with Disabilities.* Chorley: Lisieux Hall Publications.

Meisels, S.J. and Shonkoff, J.P. (Eds.) 2000. *Handbook of Early Childhood Intervention. 2nd Edition.* Cambridge: Cambridge University Press.

Miles, S., 2005. *A position paper on inclusive education.* London: Leonard Cheshire International.

Mitchell, R., 1999a. The research base of community-based rehabilitation. *Disability and Rehabilitation,* 21, 459-468.

Mitchell, R., 1999b. Community-based rehabilitation: the generalized model. *Disability and Rehabilitation,* 21, 522-528.

Neville, M., Baylis, L., Boldison, S.J., Cox, A., Cox, L., Gilliand, D., Laird, M., McIver, B. and Williams, C., 2000. *Building Inclusive Communities.* Rugby: Circles Network.

Oliver, M., 1990. *The Politics of Disablement.* London: Macmillan.

O'Toole, B., 1995. Mobilising Communities. In B.J. O'Toole, B. & R. McConkey (eds.) *Innovations in Developing Countries for People with Disabilities.* Chorley, Lancs.: Lisieux Hall Publications.

Sanderson, S., Kilbane, J. and Gitsham, N., 2000. *Person-centred planning (PCP): A resource Guide.* Available from: www.valuingpeople.gov.uk/documents/PCPResource.pdf.

Schalock, R.L. and. Keith, K.D., 2000. The concept of quality of life in the United States: Current research and application. In K.D. Keith & R.L. Schalock (eds.) *Cross- cultural perspectives on quality of life.* Washington: AAMR.

Simons, K., 1998. *Living support networks: An evaluation of the services provided by KeyRing.* Brighton: Pavilion Publishing.

Skogmo, P., 1995. Fostering the formation of parents' associations. In B.J. O'Toole, B. & R. McConkey (eds.) *Innovations in Developing Countries for People with Disabilities*. Chorley, Lancs.: Lisieux Hall Publications.

Stubbs, S., 1994. *A critical review of the literature relating to the education of disabled children in developing countries*. London: Save the Children Fund.

Swain, J., Finkelstein, V., French, S. and Oliver, M., 1993. *Disabling Barriers – Enabling Environments*. Milton Keynes: Sage Publications and Open University.

Swain, J. and French, S., 2000. Towards an affirmation model of disability. *Disability and Society*, 15, 569-582.

Thorburn, M. and Marfo, K., 1990. *Practical approaches to childhood disability in developing countries: Insights from experience and research*. St John's: Memorial University of Newfoundland.

Turmusani, M., Vreede, A. and Wirz, S., 2002. Some ethical issues in community-based rehabilitation initiatives in developing countries. *Disability and Rehabilitation*, 24, 558-564.

United Nations, 1994a. *The Standard Rules on the equalization of opportunities for persons with disabilities*. New York: UN.

United Nations, 1994b. *Community-Based Rehabilitation for and with People with Disabilities*. New York: International Labour Organization (ILO), United Nations Educational, Scientific and Cultural Organization (UNESCO) and World Health Organization (WHO).

Vanier, J., 1991. *Community and Growth*. London: Longman and Todd.

Werner, D., 1995. Strengthening the role of disabled people in community-based rehabilitation programmes. In B.J. O'Toole, B. & R. McConkey (eds.) *Innovations in Developing Countries for People with Disabilities*. Chorley, Lancs.: Lisieux Hall Publications.

World Health Organisation, 2001. *International Classification of Functioning, Disability and Health*, Geneva, WHO.

Zollers, N.J., Ramanathan, A. and Yu. M., 1999. The relationship between school culture and inclusion: how an inclusive culture supports inclusive education. *Qualitative Studies in Education*, 12, 157-174.

CHAPTER 3

INCLUSIVE EDUCATION

SUSIE MILES

I. CONCEPTS AND DEFINITIONS – DEVELOPING A LANGUAGE OF INCLUSION

There is considerable confusion associated with the term inclusive education. Definitions of the term differ according to the particular interests and concerns of organisations. Some of these definitions can be found in Appendix 2. Many practitioners have called for consistency in the use of language. This is extremely difficult, however, when the term is interpreted differently according to context and culture.

A great deal of the documents written about inclusive education come from advocacy organisations, rather than from researchers. It is therefore difficult to locate evidence which shows how inclusive approaches can be sustained and what their consequences are for learners, and disabled learners in particular. Such research is taking place primarily, though not exclusively, in Northern English speaking countries, but very little research has taken place in the South. In this section a selection of definitions of inclusive education are presented and discussed.

"Inclusive education starts from the belief that the right to education is a basic human right and the foundation for a more just society.

Inclusive education takes the Education for All (EFA) agenda forward by finding ways of enabling schools to serve all children in their communities as part of an inclusive education system.

Inclusive education is concerned with all learners, with a focus on those who have traditionally been excluded from educational opportunities – such as learners with special needs and disabilities, children from ethnic and linguistic minorities".

UNESCO, 2001a

The quotation above is taken from the 'Open File on Inclusive Education: Support Materials for Managers and Administrators'. See Appendix 2 for further quotations from the Open File. These materials were developed over many years by practitioners from a wide range of countries. UNESCO has had a major influence on the development of inclusive education internationally and has produced many documents for those seeking to develop more inclusive practices in schools. These materials are informed by research on an inclusive approach to school improvement. This approach is based on clearly stated values, reflecting a social model of disability. The emphasis in most UNESCO publications is on the need for system change and on the right to access quality education. Including children from marginalised groups is seen as an issue of social justice and anti-discrimination, but also as an opportunity for education systems to embrace change.

This approach to inclusive education recognises that pupils experience difficulties because of the ways in which schools are organised and the way teaching is provided. It is therefore argued that schools need to be reformed and pedagogy improved so that schools can respond positively to pupil diversity – seeing individual differences not as problems to be fixed, but as opportunities for enriching learning. (See figures 1 and 2 on page 71. They are taken from "Learning from Difference", an EENET action research report (Miles et al, 2003), but were developed in the late 1990s by Save the Children disability advisers.

SPECIAL EDUCATIONAL NEEDS

The term *special educational needs* was first developed in the UK over 20 years ago following the Warnock report of 1978 (Department of Education and Sciences, 1978), has been widely adopted and tends to be used without any clear definition. Children with 'special educational needs' is often used to mean children with disabilities. Yet not all disabled children have special needs, and not all children with special educational needs have disabilities.

The field of 'special needs' and inclusive education is full of contradiction and confusion. Some of this confusion has arisen because of the tendency of Southern countries to look to the North for ideas on how to educate disabled children and those identified as having 'special needs'. Many Northern agencies have also encouraged Southern governments to adopt models of service provision, such as special units attached to mainstream schools, which may work well in highly resourced situations, but tend not to work so well where there are limited material resources.

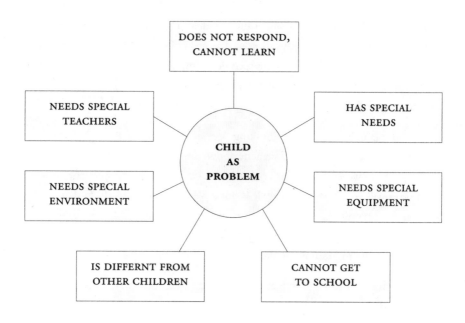

Figure1: Individual differences as the problem

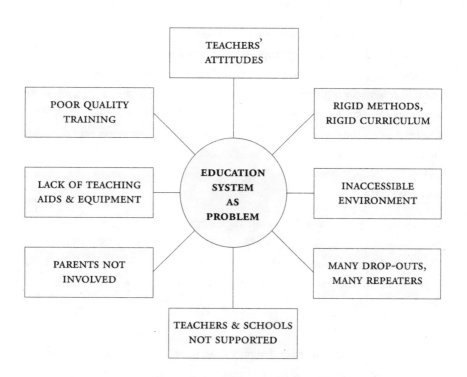

Figure 2: The system as the problem

The term *special education* is sometimes used as a general term summarising a variety of approaches to the education of disabled children and those experiencing difficulties in learning. Yet for many people it implies segregated learning and is often seen as being in opposition to inclusive education. Still special schools and specialist staff can have a vital role to play in promoting inclusive education.

In promoting inclusion and re-thinking *special needs education*, it is important that we move towards some agreement about the meaning of key terms. This is challenging, however, as inclusive education is a continuing process, and so definitions will continually change. It is not a fixed state, or something that can be achieved by a certain date. Understanding inclusion as a process enables us to move beyond arguments 'for' or 'against' inclusive education. Instead, the issue is about working together to promote progress.

See Appendix 2 for some examples of the wide range of interpretations of the term inclusive education by international non-governmental organisations, the UK government and UNESCO.

2. HISTORY OF INCLUSIVE EDUCATION

This section reviews the key international agreements signed over the last 15 years which have provided an impetus to the promotion of inclusive education internationally. This does not mean that inclusive education only began in 1990, but it highlights the fact that the right to education for all groups of children became a more prominent international issue. See Appendix 3 for a summary of the UN Convention on the Rights of the Child and the World Conferences on Education for All which took place in Jomtien in 1990 and Dakar in 2000.

SALAMANCA

One of the most influential international agreements was "The Salamanca Statement on Principles, Policy and Practice in Special Needs Education" (UNESCO, 1994). The World Conference on Special Needs Education was held in Salamanca in 1994 between the conferences in Jomtien and Dakar. Its main aim was to further the objectives of Education for All (EFA). It provides a framework and guidance on developing inclusive education internationally:

- Education systems should be designed and educational programmes implemented to take into account the wide diversity of characteristics and needs.

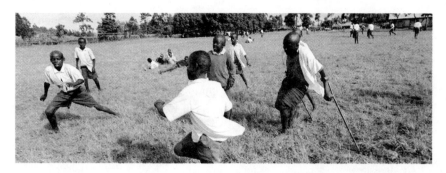

- Those who have special educational needs must have access to regular schools which should accommodate them within a child-centred pedagogy capable of meeting these needs.

Many practitioners argue that the Salamanca Statement is one of the most significant international documents influencing inclusive education. Yet its influence remains within the 'special needs' world and these documents tend not to be widely known or quoted within the wider context of EFA. Katerina Tomasevski, the UN Rapporteur on the Right to Education, has severely criticised Salamanca:

> "The Salamanca Statement has more or less collapsed because it was strong on nouns like empowerment, inclusion and quality education but extremely weak on who has the obligation to do what. As a result the key part of human rights strategy which is challenging violations and denials of human rights has been prevented from happening." (Tomasevski, 2004, p5)

Nevertheless Salamanca has proved to be a useful reference point in the recent debates about the new UN Convention on Disability. In their protests against the apparent move back to more segregated forms of educational provision, campaigners for inclusive education have called for a return to the 'principles enshrined in Salamanca'.

Salamanca has undoubtedly been helpful in encouraging some practitioners and policy makers to look at educational difficulties in new ways. This new direction in thinking is based on the belief that changes in methodology and organisation made in response to pupils experiencing difficulties can, under certain conditions, benefit all children. In this way, pupils who are currently categorised as having special needs come to be seen as a stimulus for encouraging the development of richer and more child-friendly learning environments.

Although there is some evidence of progress in developing inclusive education in a wide range of different contexts, it is far from easy; progress is still limited in most countries and not all practitioners are comfortable with an inclusive philosophy.

Inclusive policies and practices should be unique to the context in which they are developed. It is important to remember that a range of inclusive possibilities can be considered:

> ".... it seems to me mistaken to look for a single set of policies or practices which will somehow 'deliver' inclusive education. Such policies and practices have to be developed in different contexts to address whatever threats to equity arise in different systems, at different times and for different groups of children". (Dyson, 2004, p.615)

In countries where education is not compulsory, it is not only disabled children who are denied access to schooling. Furthermore alternative and indigenous forms of education are often considered valuable, especially when formal schooling simply is not an option. This may be the case for working children, 'street' children, children from nomadic families, as well as for disabled children. United Nations conventions and international statements have to be interpreted in a wide range of different contexts, but are often written with a bias towards Western ideas about education.

By implication, inclusive education can take many different forms, depending on the context in which it is implemented and on the definition of the term in that context. It is argued in this paper that inclusive education is not a fixed state, but part of the process of moving towards a more inclusive society. It cannot therefore be neatly packaged as a single policy.

THE MILLENNIUM DEVELOPMENT GOALS

The new international targets outlined in the Millennium Development Goals (MDGs) include access to and completion of Universal Primary Education by 2015. However, if marginalised groups of learners, such as those with disabilities, continue to be excluded from primary education, it will not be possible for countries to achieve the MDG on education. National plans to achieve universal primary education tend to be implemented independently of any inclusive education initiatives.

Even in the context of the most committed approach to EFA, systems still exclude vulnerable groups of children from educational opportunities, so there is an urgent need for an inclusive approach to EFA.

"The question is often asked why inclusive education is necessary as a new educational strategy, particularly in those countries that have a commitment to and apparent existing policies on education for all...Will the adoption of a strategy to build more inclusive education systems and institutions help or hinder the achievement of the very urgent and important objective of EFA? The answer is emphatic. Without the development of inclusive policies in education ....EFA will not be achieved." (UNESCO, 2001b)

Some organisations see inclusive education as being solely an issue related to disabled learners. A key reason for this seems to be a focus on the need for specialist resources in the development of educational provision for children identified as having disabilities and/or special educational needs.

An inclusive approach to EFA does not mean that there would be no access to specialist support for disabled learners. Is it realistic, however, in the context of the South, to develop a separate special education system first, and then progress towards more inclusive provision? This 'stages' approach reflects the historical development of special education in the North in the twentieth century, but does not necessarily provide a blueprint for progress towards EFA in the South in the twenty-first century.

Clearly EFA requires additional resources; an inclusive approach to EFA will require resources to develop access to specialist support for some disabled children; and a lack of resources does present a barrier. Nevertheless, the question remains of how resources should be prioritised and whether they can be more creatively used to promote inclusive education in the context of EFA.

In response to concerns that Education for All initiatives do not necessarily include disabled children, UNESCO has worked with international disability-focused organisations to establish an EFA *Flagship* entitled, "The Right to Education for Persons with Disabilities: Towards Inclusion". Its main goal is to ensure that national EFA plans incorporate disabled people. Other flagships exist to highlight the particular issues of gender, HIV/AIDS, teacher education, and so on. The Flagship was a response to the perceived lack of attention given to disabled children at Dakar in 2000.

Inclusive education is increasingly seen as being part of an inclusive approach to international development by organisations such as DfID, the International Disability and Development Consortium and the World Bank.

The challenge of ensuring that disabled children and those categorised as having special educational needs gain access to education and *successfully complete* their primary school education is considerable – but it is achievable. We have the knowledge, but it will depend upon whether national governments have the will to make it happen.

Statistics are notoriously unreliable on this issue because of the differences in definition of 'disability' and 'special needs' across cultures and contexts. The figure of two per cent is often put forward as the number of disabled children who attend school in Southern countries, leaving 98% out of school. Yet anecdotal evidence indicates that as many as 50% of some groups of disabled children may be attending school. Progress is extremely patchy.

3. LEONARD CHESHIRE INTERNATIONAL

LCI offers support for programme design and management, professional and community training, campaign and policy development. The organisation works with disability partner organisations focusing on key areas in the life of people with disabilities, including early years, practical support with every day life, inclusive education and economic empowerment.

The main themes in the inclusive education work include:

- Development, documentation and replication of a model of inclusive education;
- Establishment of partnerships with ministries of education for teacher training and curricula improvement;
- Provision of training to primary school teachers on detection and appropriate didactic methodologies;
- Promotion of improvement of schools' physical environments;
- Provision of training and support for parents;
- Promotion of meaningful education for disabled children and effective monitoring of impact.

Case study in Kenya

The key features of the work in Oriang include:

- A pilot programme implemented in partnership with the Ministry of Education of Kenya targeting five primary schools in the Kisumu District;

- Involvement of families and the communities in school management and mobilisation;
- A focus on economic empowerment;
- A tested and documented model to be scaled up in other locations.

Case study in Malawi

This is a much smaller initiative than the one in Oriang. It involves:

- Awareness raising and advocacy for education rights of disabled children targeting communities and the Ministry of Education;
- Working in partnership with the Commonwealth Education Fund and UNICEF.

4. KEY ISSUES

This section focuses on ten issues facing practitioners and policy makers as they promote and implement inclusive education in a range of different contexts. Examples are provided of inclusive practices in a range of countries, including the experience of Leonard Cheshire International. The examples simply highlight some of the key issues for Southern countries and should be seen as a source of inspiration and an opportunity for reflection, rather than as a blueprint for inclusion:

> "[it is not] the case that some countries have discovered the secret of inclusion and should be held up as shining examples for the rest of us to follow. Instead, we each have to maintain a constant vigilance in our own situations, learning what we can from each other, offering help and guidance, but not imposing solutions that may well not work in different contexts." (Dyson, 2004, p.615)

There are some general principles and assumptions which underpin this discussion paper on inclusive education. The first is a commitment to carrying out a comprehensive situation analysis prior to implementation. Linked to this is the importance of identifying and building on local resources and initiatives. It is also acknowledged that ideally there should be shared ownership of inclusive education programmes between schools, families and communities. Education is not seen as a separate entity; it is only one aspect of the life of a disabled child, and is not necessarily the primary concern of families and carers, especially if the child is severely disabled.

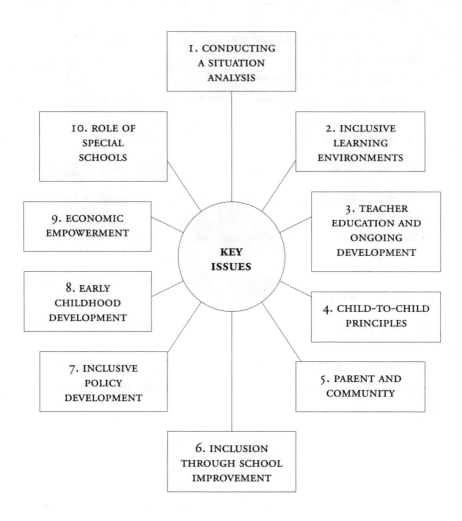

Figure 3: Key issues in inclusive education

As the Oriang example shows, it is important to develop a pilot school, or a cluster of pilot schools, as a model of inclusive education and a focus for learning. It is important, though, that a careful plan is developed to ensure that there is progression from the pilot school to other schools in the country. Good leadership is essential.

Ideally training should be provided to mainstream school teachers through short in-service courses, based in schools and in the community. Inevitably there is a need to re-orient the role of special educators towards working in inclusive settings. Locating specialist support at district and national levels, rather than at school level, will help to sustain an inclusive and equitable system. This can be problematic, however, when distances are great and transport facilities are limited. Locating specialist support at school level is an unaffordable option for many education systems. Besides, inclusive education aims to benefit all children, not only children with disabilities. Success depends to a large extent on the careful and planned use of existing resources.

Each of the key issues is illustrated with examples from schools and communities. The challenges and implications for practitioners are also discussed. Figure 3 neatly summarises the key issues and provides a reference point for readers.

4.1 SITUATION ANALYSIS

Issue: *an important starting point in promoting inclusive education is to carry out a situation analysis which identifies existing resources and initiatives and highlights the way forward.*

Quito, Ecuador

In 2005 the Fundacion General Ecuatoriana, the organisation of disabled people and one of LCI's partners, initiated a pilot research study to evaluate the progress of integrated education in Ecuador. The aim of the study is to identify effective teaching and learning practices and the gaps in provision.

The results of the study will provide the foundations for the design of an inclusive education pilot project.

Oriang, Kenya

In 1999 a situational needs analysis was undertaken in partnership with representatives of the local community. Local partners identified the need for disabled children to attend school and for schools to be supported to become more inclusive. It was this initiative that led to the setting up of the Inclusive Education programme.

In analysing a country situation it is important to identify the key players. In the example from Ecuador, LCI worked with both the Ministry of Education and the disabled people's organisation. Identifying the key players can be a time-consuming process. However it is time and money well spent, and the document which is produced through the situation analysis process becomes valuable baseline information as the programme is implemented.

Key challenges

- How can practitioners be supported to conduct their own situation analyses in order to reduce the dependency on external consultants?
- How can regions be supported to develop their own expertise, and an appreciation of the key issues in that region?

4.2 INCLUSIVE LEARNING ENVIRONMENTS

Issue: *learning environments tend not to be conducive to learning or to the inclusion of disabled children. Architects continue to build inaccessible school buildings.*

Creating a welcoming and accessible environment in which children can learn is a major part of inclusive education. Children need to be able to travel safely to school and be in a safe physical and social environment. They also need a caring and stimulating learning environment to understand what is being taught and be able to interact with their peers and teachers. This may require the adjustment of teaching methods, materials, settings and timetabling, instead of adjusting the children to existing methods. Such adjustments will benefit education quality for all children – not only those with a disability.

Possible strategies drawn from the work of Save the Children, UK (2002) include:

- Use simple, clear and consistent language;
- Make learning enjoyable and fun;
- Promote active learning;
- Make education more relevant to daily life and home situations;
- Accept that children learn at different rates and vary teaching methods accordingly;
- Respond flexibly and creatively to the individual needs of children;
- Be flexible about seating arrangements – use mats, wooden blocks or old car tyres;
- Ensure that children can see, hear and understand;
- Encourage teachers to observe each other and problem-solve together;
- Involve parents and community members in education.

It is not only the physical environment which needs to be made more inclusive. Teaching and learning styles can be adapted so that they are accessible to all. Creating a welcoming and accessible physical environment complements good teaching.

Oriang, Kenya

Leonard Cheshire International has been supporting a pilot inclusive education programme in five schools in Oriang, Western Kenya. The project benefits 2,200 children of whom approximately 10% have minor to severe disabilities. There has been a strong focus on making the school environment more inclusive, both in teaching and learning styles and in terms of the physical environment. Physical adaptations have included:

- building ramps
- constructing accessible toilets
- enlarging classroom windows
- painting walls white to improve lighting
- repairing classrooms
- levelling playgrounds

See Compass Issue 20 (LC, 2004) and Enabling Education Issue 8 (Ogot, 2004) for further information.

A physically accessible environment is an important component in creating welcoming and inclusive environments in which all children can learn. Although it is not a substitute for good quality teaching and learning, it is nevertheless an aspect of inclusive education which is often overlooked. In Oriang this has involved the buiding of ramps, lowering blackboards and widening doorways which help wheelchair users.

The Oriang example is breaking new ground in the way that it has addressed a whole range of environmental issues. For example, the issue of inaccessible and poorly maintained school sanitation is a major one for the majority of the world's school children – not only for disabled learners. It is a major contributing factor to the high drop-out rate among teenage girls in many African countries, for example. The Oriang schools have built accessible toilets demonstrating their commitment to developing inclusive environments. However unforeseen difficulties with shortages of water, hygiene, and paths, which are frequently washed away by the rain, are some examples of the ongoing challenges.

The quality of light inside the classroom can have a major impact on the quality and accessibility of teaching and learning. The Oriang schools have painted the classroom walls white and enlarged their windows. Windows in African classrooms tend to be small because glass is unaffordable and they keep the rain out, but the

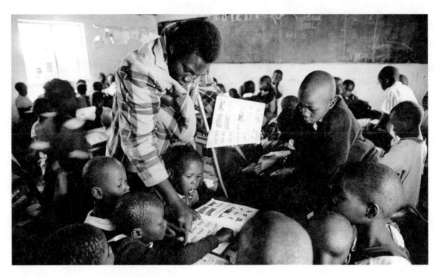

Photo: Gideon Mendel / Leonard Cheshire

large windows have proved to be problematic in the rainy season. This is an issue which deserves more attention in discussions about accessible school architecture and educational inclusion.

Key challenges

- How can inclusive learning environments be promoted using locally available resources?
- How can governments and international agencies be influenced to design accessible teaching and learning environments?

4.3 TEACHER EDUCATION AND ONGOING DEVELOPMENT

Issue: *Teachers are arguably the most valuable human resources available to promote inclusive practices. If they do not believe in inclusion, they can become a major barrier to progress. In many cases teachers lack confidence and the basic knowledge needed to welcome all children into their classes.*

Teachers often think they need 'special skills' to teach disabled children, but experience has shown that in most cases disabled children can be included through good, clear and accessible teaching which encourages the active participation of children. These are all skills which teachers need to deliver quality education to all children, disabled or non-disabled. In addition to these skills, teachers may also need some specific technical help and/or equipment to meet the needs of some children.

Honduras

In Honduras, Leonard Cheshire and Fundación Casayuda are in the process of launching an innovative inclusive education project. Teachers from both special and inclusive schools are being trained to respond positively to student diversity. Casayuda's teachers have received training from Leonard Cheshire in arts-based approaches to facilitate inclusive education. The Leonard Cheshire regional office, with the collaboration of its partner organisation in Ecuador, Fundacion General Ecuatoriana (FGE), facilitated a training workshop for the teachers participating in the pilot project, Ministry of Education staff, and NGOs working in the field. This is not only a training programme, but it is also a form of regional information sharing between Honduras and Ecuador. Training material has been drawn from a range of training packs available internationally. See Appendix 4 for details of Training Packs.

Zambia

In the Mpika Inclusive Education Programme, there were only a small number of teachers who had special training. The Mpika teachers were used to meeting regularly to share experiences and solve their problems, both within individual schools and between clusters of schools. With the support of the teachers responsible for providing in-service training, the teachers have gained confidence in their own local expertise and have developed their own locally appropriate solutions. Previously they had relied on specialist teachers to work with children identified as having special educational needs and disabilities (Miles et al, 2003).

Laos

Teachers receive a short initial training course of 3-5 days. They are then provided with lots of follow-up support and monitoring. In this way they are able to learn by doing. Their tutors can adopt a problem-based learning approach, using real situations in classrooms as opportunities for professional development, rather than simply delivering a theoretical curriculum. The teachers are able to share their experiences and find mutual solutions through a newsletter.

An action research approach to teacher development

Action research methods can be used to involve key stakeholders in asking critical questions about inclusive education in their context. EENET has been involved in an action research project focusing on inclusive education in Zambia and Tanzania, funded by DFID. In both countries it was assumed that specially trained teachers had the sole responsibility for inclusive education. The term 'inclusive education' was associated with the teaching of children identified as having special educational needs, or disabilities, and was often used interchangeably with the terms 'special' or 'integrated education'.

Referring to 'inclusive education' as 'the process of addressing barriers to the presence, participation and achievement of all children in their local neighbourhood schools', encouraged both mainstream and specialist teachers to think differently about the meaning of inclusion. They adopted a 'barrier analysis' approach to the promotion of inclusive education in schools and communities, which can enable practitioners to adopt a broader approach to educational exclusion. They asked questions about who was not present in school and why, and who was not participating, and therefore not achieving, in school. This process revealed many different groups of learners who were not present and not participating, including girls who had heavy domestic workloads or who had been married at an early age, boys who were more interested in street culture than learning, children affected by HIV/AIDS, as well as children with a range of disabilities. Teachers from a cluster of schools were encouraged to reflect on their own practice and to write about the particular challenges they faced in promoting inclusion. The Zambian teachers' stories are on EENET's web site (www.eenet.org.uk) and the publication is called 'Researching Our Experience'.

Since teachers are such an important human resource in transforming education systems, it is essential that an inclusive approach to teacher education is adopted. Teachers need ongoing support and development and the type of training offered in most countries desperately needs to be transformed. Influencing teacher educators is therefore a key issue in implementing inclusive education.

Ideally change should be introduced at the level of pre-service teacher education, but this cannot be done successfully in a college, away from the reality of classrooms. Trainee teachers need to see examples of inclusion in action, and so ideally pilot projects should be developed in order to provide teachers with relevant experience. Finally the roles of specialist teachers and specialist teacher educators need to be re-oriented so that they can adapt their skills to an inclusive educational system.

The payment of teachers' salaries is the biggest single item in any school budget in both income-rich and income-poor countries. Teachers are therefore the biggest single human resource which requires training. Ongoing teacher education is costly and can be difficult 'logistically in countries with a poor infrastructure and a large rural population. Building teachers' confidence and encouraging teacher-to-teacher support are two ways in which progress towards inclusive education can be made.

Key challenges

- How can teachers be supported to respond appropriately to diversity in their classrooms?
- How can teacher education materials be developed which reflect the realities of promoting inclusive practices?

4.4 CHILD-TO-CHILD PRINCIPLES

Issue: *Children can play a role in their own education and in the education of their peers. In the context of large class sizes and over-worked teachers, children are a valuable human resource.*

The communication of key health messages by older children to their younger siblings is a strategy pioneered by the Child-to-Child Trust since the 1970s. However, child-to-child methodologies have only been used relatively recently by educationalists to promote inclusive practices. Yet they have great potential to bring about changes in attitude and in mobilising the often under-utilised human resource of large numbers of children.

Zambia

In Mpika, Zambia, there is a very strong history of teachers communicating health education messages through child-to-child methods, and of the activities being incorporated into maths, English, geography and social studies lessons. In the mid-1990s they began to use the same methods to explore community attitudes to disability. School children were asked to conduct a community survey to identify those children who were 'out of school', and to find out why they stayed at home. This was very successful in raising awareness and in including children in school who would otherwise have remained at home. It was also a very effective way of encouraging the parents of some of the children to reduce their domestic workloads to enable them to attend school. A project was then developed to break down the social barriers which existed between the children being educated in the special unit and those in the main school. The focus was on developing friendships, travelling to school together, home visits at weekends, providing support with academic work etc. More information about Child-to-Child is available from: www.childtochild.org

---

Children are an important and valuable human resource – especially in communities where there is a high death rate among teachers as a result of the impact of HIV/AIDS. Children can play an effective role in promoting inclusion while at the same time learning about social justice and human rights. Teachers often lack confidence, however, in working with children in this way, especially in school systems which have a strong authoritarian approach, and in cultures where children tend not to challenge adults' opinions.

Key challenges

- How can children take more responsibility for their own education?
- How can children be encouraged to take responsibility for their peers?
- How can CBR workers and teachers work together more closely to promote Child-to-Child activities?

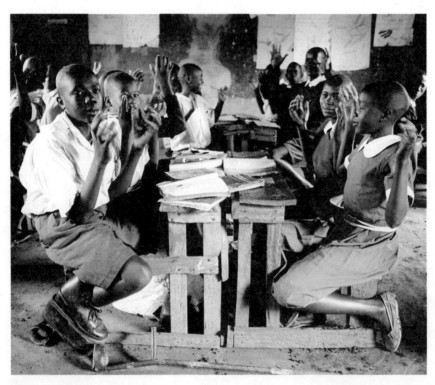

Photo: Gideon Mendel / Leonard Cheshire

4.5 Parent and community involvement

Issue: *Families and communities are a valuable human resource with an important role to play in their children's education.*

It has often been said that the countries which have made the most progress towards inclusion in education are those countries with strong parents' organisations which have campaigned for their children to be included. Parental involvement in their children's education is a key factor in educational progress. It is even more important for those children who are vulnerable to exclusion and who have impairments which make learning more challenging. Parent-teacher communication and collaboration is therefore crucial, yet it is difficult to achieve.

There are many examples around the world of highly successful parent-led initiatives, many of which have become well-established professionally-led organisations. A key issue for parents is whether they should remain as advocates, or whether they should be drawn into service provision because they want schools for their children today and can't afford to wait until their advocacy has achieved its goals tomorrow.

'Family Action for Inclusion in Education'

In 1999 EENET began a process of collecting stories written by parents' organisations. The stories from South Africa, Lesotho, Nepal, India, Romania, Australia and the UK were made available on the web site in 2001. In the following year EENET produced a publication based on these stories as a resource for new parents' organisations wishing to influence change. It has been widely used in many countries, including by a disabled person's organisation in the UK, to convince teachers of the valuable role parents can play. There are many common threads between the Northern and Southern stories – in both contexts the parents expressed their need to talk to other parents of disabled children and to recruit others to join them. In Australia and South Africa the parents organised demonstrations to demand that the rights of their children be respected by the governments. However there were also some important differences. In the UK the parents organised around one particular impairment and ethnic group, while in Lesotho there was a broad membership including all disabilities and the organisation felt it was important to take a broader look at exclusion and to play a key role nationally in campaigning for the rights of all children.

Parents have a key role to play in supporting their children and in campaigning for inclusive education. Like children, they are a valuable human resource which is often overlooked by educators. Parents play a valuable role as part of community based committees in supporting the inclusive education programme in Oriang, Kenya. The following case studies of individual children illustrate the importance of a close working relationship between schools, families and their communities.

Case Studies

Gloria is a young girl of 7 years who has six sisters. Her mother is a widow and is supported by a Community Assistant Chief. Her livelihood depends on the small farm left behind by her husband, where she grows potatoes, bananas and maize for domestic use.

Gloria was born at home in 1997, assisted by a village midwife. She was a healthy baby, but developed a fever with convulsions. She was taken to a local health centre and was treated for malaria. Two years later she had another fever and severe convulsions. This time she was diagnosed with epilepsy, as the convulsions lasted for more than seven hours.

One of the officials from the Leonard Cheshire Inclusive Education Programme met Gloria's mother at a Chief's baraza (meeting) in which he explained about the project. Since then a Community Health Worker has been visiting the girl to ensure she is provided with the required medication. The project team takes her to the district hospital when she develops severe convulsions and fits. Currently Oriang' Inclusive Education staff are making arrangements to train a local nurse at the Mission Dispensary to dispense epileptic drugs and to assist community members identified with epilepsy.

Samuel is the first born in a family of seven. His father is a teacher and his mother is a housewife – both parents take full responsibility for him. Samuel was born a healthy baby in 1993, but at the age of 8 he began to have convulsions. His parents noticed that his right limbs were becoming weak, and his body was trembling. The parents took Samuel to the district hospital where the doctors treated him for malaria but there was no response so they started treatment for meningitis. He was hospitalised for two months and since then he has had a physical disability and speech problems. Through the Community Health Workers, Samuel has been given exercises, and provided with a sitting/standing aid. Members of the Inclusive Education programme staff have taught the parents how to assist him at home.

Key challenges

- How can parents become more involved in their children's education?

- How can teachers be encouraged to involve parents in their children's education?

- Is it appropriate for parents to be involved in service provision?

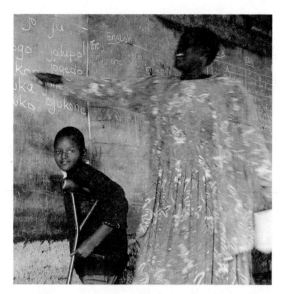

Photo: Gideon Mendel / Leonard Cheshire

4.6 INCLUSION THROUGH SCHOOL IMPROVEMENT

Issue: *there is a need to improve the quality of education for all children. The experience of educating disabled children can, in some cases, bring new insights to the school improvement challenge.*

"School improvement may be a result of inclusive education, or it may provide the opportunity for more inclusive practices to be promoted. Whichever route is taken, school improvement must take place". Save the Children UK, 2002

Laos

Save the Children UK was asked by the government of the Laos People's Democratic Republic in 1989 to assist with pre- and in-service teacher training as part of a large-scale school improvement programme. Research in classrooms revealed that very little attention was paid to individual learning needs. A discussion of children's learning needs and appropriate strategies to respond to them led naturally to the integrated education programme in primary schools and later in the kindergarten. In this way a school improvement programme laid the foundations for inclusive education.

School improvement can help prepare schools for an inclusive education programme. It is also possible for inclusive education to lead the way for school improvement to take place.

Improving the quality of education for all

Education cannot be inclusive without being good quality, and the reverse is also true: education cannot be good quality without being inclusive. Good quality education is:

- responsive
- relevant
- developmentally appropriate and
- participatory.

This is also true of inclusive education. Including all children involves challenging discrimination and prejudice, building on children's strengths, and using child-centred approaches. Inclusive education can act as a catalyst for change in educational practice, leading to improved quality of education. Including disabled children in mainstream schools challenges teachers to develop more child-centred, participatory, and active teaching approaches – and this benefits all children.

Inclusive education has been introduced in many countries with modest education budgets, and relatively little technical help. Improvements in teaching quality and student achievement (as well as reduced drop-out and failure rates), have been some of the positive outcomes. For example, anecdotal evidence from Lesotho, Zambia and Laos indicates that inclusive approaches can improve academic achievement. Teachers in Lesotho also reported that they had become 'better teachers'. However no systematic data has been collected to demonstrate the wider benefits of inclusion for the whole education system.

Key challenges

- How can schools be supported to become better schools for all children?
- How can teachers gain confidence in their ability to teach all children?
- How can schools be supported over time to provide quality, inclusive education to all children, including those with disabilities?

4.7 INCLUSIVE POLICY DEVELOPMENT

Issue: *inclusive education is seen by policy makers as a version of special education and so it is not a mainstream issue.*

> "The key challenge is to ensure that the broad vision of EFA as an inclusive concept is reflected in national government and funding agency policies."
> Dakar Framework for Action on EFA, para 19

The major international documents such as the UN's Standard Rules, Convention on the Rights of the Child, and the Salamanca and Dakar Frameworks all indicate that disabled children have a right to education. Some go further and state clearly that they have the right to attend their neighbourhood school. Yet very few national policy documents make this clear. Too often the issue of 'special needs education' is seen as something separate, and so is marginalised from the main education policy.

Tegusigalpa, Honduras

In 1997 the Special Education Department in Honduras was closed in an effort to introduce inclusion following the Salamanca Conference. Unfortunately the closure of this department did not lead to more inclusive initiatives. However the department has re-opened with a new director of Special Education who is working as part of a team of three people to 'mainstream' inclusive education within EFA initiatives. The impetus to work inclusively is partly due to the fact that there are no separate funds available to work separately, but also because the new Director is committed to an inclusive way of working.

It is essential to incorporate the educational needs of disabled children into national EFA action plans and to ensure that an inclusive approach to EFA is adopted at country level.

Key challenges

- How can EFA initiatives be supported to become more inclusive of all children?
- How can inclusive education policies be developed while at the same time ensuring that disabled children have access to a quality education?

4.8 EARLY CHILDHOOD DEVELOPMENT

Issue: *Early childhood development can reduce the disabling effects of impairments and should form an integral part of inclusive education programmes.*

One of the major differences between educational provision in the North and South is the attention paid to early childhood development in the North which helps to reduce the disabling effects of impairments and provide children with the best possible start in life. In addition, the principles of early childhood education have a great deal in common with those of special education: practical active learning with lots of reinforcement and repetition. Intervention in the early years can make an enormous difference to the rest of the child's life.

Brazil

In conjunction with local education authorities, Cheshire Brazil converted a former residential home for people with disabilities into an inclusive preschool for children from poor families, many of whom are disabled. The project is being carried out in conjunction with the government social-aid and education departments, who want to maximise the limited resources available to the children's families. The desperate need for early years provision was a major motivating factor in this dramatic change in Brazil.

In many countries early years provision continues to be overlooked and under-prioritised. Pre-school classes, where they exist, are often over-subscribed and in a poor state of repair. Yet inclusive early childhood education can lay the foundation for lifelong inclusion in both education and society. Sadly, most inclusive education initiatives focus exclusively on primary education, in line with the international focus on universal access to, and completion of, primary education.

Key challenges

- How can capacity in early years provision be developed to support inclusive education programmes?

- How can inclusive education programmes work more effectively with CBR programmes to ensure that disabled children are identified at an early age and provided with opportunities for inclusive early childhood education?

4.9 ECONOMIC EMPOWERMENT

Issue: *inclusive education cannot be implemented in isolation poverty reduction and economic empowerment are key to the success of inclusive education programmes.*

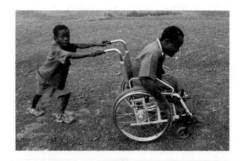

Photo: Jenny Matthews / Leonard Cheshire

Disability and poverty are inextricably linked. Poor children are less likely to receive early intervention and support, and more likely to suffer lasting impairments. The reverse is also true: families struggling with disability are more likely to be trapped in poverty due to a range of challenges including negative attitudes, problems with mobility, earning power, child-care, etc. Children and families struggling with disability are systematically excluded, and the poorer they are, the greater that exclusion is likely to be. Being included in education can help disabled children to break out of the cycle of poverty and exclusion.

The provision of school meals is one of the possible responses to poverty in many countries, although it is often unaffordable or impractical where water supplies are unreliable. Where there is a large number of children receiving free school meals in England, there tends also to be a large number of children identified as having special educational needs, or being 'at risk'. Free school meals is one of the indicators of poverty and social disadvantage.

Oriang, Kenya

At the LCI regional meeting in Kisumu in 2004 a discussion was held about the links between economic empowerment and inclusive education. In order to support the sustainability of the community involvement initiative in implementing inclusive education in Oriang, it was agreed that economic empowerment programmes should also be introduced. In particular, there is a need to address the poor conditions in which some children are living in Oriang, and the fact that many come to school hungry and poorly clothed.

Key challenges

* How can inclusive education programmes respond to the challenge of poverty and social exclusion?

4.10 ROLE OF SPECIAL SCHOOLS

Issue: *there is an unhelpful polarisation between those who believe in promoting special schools and those who seek to promote inclusive practices – yet the majority of disabled children do not attend school at all.*

Some have argued that progress towards a more inclusive education system poses a challenge to special education as it has developed over the last 20 years or so. However inclusive education is far more complex than the debate about 'mainstream or special':

"It is simply not the case that inclusion would be achieved if all countries closed their special schools and placed disabled children in regular classes". Dyson, 2004

Currently the UK government is concerned to debate how those working within the special education system, and those working within mainstream schools, can collaborate in developing more inclusive practices. In this regard, the expertise of those working within special schools will be seen as a resource for inclusion and will not be disregarded. A continued role for special schools in the UK context has been suggested through, for example:

- Sharing expertise with mainstream schools to support greater inclusion
- Promoting greater staff and pupil movement between mainstream and special school sectors
- Encouraging special schools to participate in federation, cluster and twinning arrangements with mainstream schools.

We need to address the question of how to develop support structures, specialist resources and professionals for children characterised as having special educational needs – in the context of limited resources and a poorly-trained teaching force. The dilemma is that a push for inclusion without such development could result in children being inadequately supported. On the other hand, the danger of waiting until specialist resources are in place, before implementing inclusion, could mean that inclusion is never achieved. The right to access specialist resources is therefore unlikely to be achieved in the near future for many children.

However there is an increasing trend for special schools to provide an impetus to the development of inclusive education, as in the following example.

In Honduras LCI is working with an NGO, Casayuda, whose leader is a disabled person. Some years ago she opened a special school in Comayagua, the second largest city in Honduras. In collaboration with Casayuda, LCI is planning to include children from the special school into neighbouring schools. The special school will mainstream their students into the neighbouring primary schools and will become a resource centre for the support of inclusive education. It will also begin to educate children with severe disabilities that mainstream schools are unable to cater for at the moment.

Residential special schools

The placing of children away from their homes and families to attend residential special schools contravenes their rights to home, family and their involvement in the community. Although there may, sometimes, be educational benefits to attending a special school, the separation of disabled children from their families and communities often confirms society's prejudice towards disabled people.

Disabled children living in institutions are particularly vulnerable to neglect, and to physical and sexual abuse. They are more dependent on larger numbers of adults, often for quite intimate forms of care. Those children who are totally dependent on carers in daily life will be most at risk – very young and female disabled children in particular. When abuse takes place, children isolated in institutions have no one to help them complain or defend themselves.

Oriang, Kenya

Oriang Cheshire Service was set up in 1975 by a group of parents of disabled children. It began as a term-time hostel (not a residential special school) for physically disabled children from the neighbouring districts who were attending Oriang Primary School. This service is now being re-oriented towards a community disability service which will support disabled children in the community. The hostel will gradually be phased out.

Focus on single impairment issues

There are some inevitable dilemmas and contradictions on the journey towards inclusion. One such dilemma is about balancing the needs of learners with a particular impairment with the principles endorsed in the Salamanca Statement.

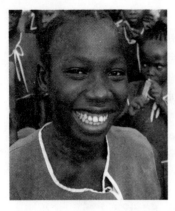

Photo: Gideon Mendel / Leonard Cheshire

'Promotion and Protection of the Rights and Dignity of Persons with Disabilities' – a new UN Convention

The draft article on education, Article 17, of the new UN Disability Convention has proved to be the most contentious of all the articles debated in New York over recent months. It has highlighted the ongoing dilemma of balancing specialist provision (in this case for deaf children, blind children and deafblind children) with more inclusive provision.

The Centre for Studies of Inclusive Education (CSIE 2004) has argued that the current draft establishes: "the segregation of disabled learners and learners with special educational needs into special schools as a legitimate human right". The CSIE "considers such a discussion to be a retrograde step in the field of education for persons with disabilities" and is lobbying for this to be reconsidered.

Inclusion International has suggested that Article 17 of the new Convention will only be acceptable to its members if it is based on the principles laid out in Salamanca.

Here are some other examples of the often delicate balance between a single impairment focus and more inclusive approaches.

The International Council for the Education of the Visually Impaired (ICEVI) – World Blind Union (WBU)

The ICEVI-WBU Discussion Paper on Inclusive Education affirms its support for Salamanca (ICEVI, 2003). It also states that special schools will continue to be promoted, whilst providing specialist support for blind children and those with low vision in the context of inclusive education.

Inclusion International is a member of the International Disability Alliance, consisting of leading international self-advocacy organisations, and is the only member organisation that involves parents. Its main focus is on children with 'intellectual impairments'. Inclusion International has taken a strong stance in support of the right of disabled children to access inclusive education by launching its own MDGs "to ensure that people with disabilities are not forgotten in global efforts to improve quality of life in developing and transitional economies."

Focus on deafness and sign language

The issue of deafness and inclusion is perhaps the most contested of all the impairment issues, as many deaf people see themselves as being members of a linguistic minority rather than as having an impairment or disability. The World Federation of the Deaf is an international campaigning group which lobbies for the right of deaf people to access sign language. Article 21 of the Salamanca Statement and Framework for Action upholds the right of deaf children to be taught in the medium of sign language.

There are, however, many challenges to achieving this, especially in income-poor countries: national sign languages need to be developed and dictionaries created, qualified teachers of deaf children are in short supply, signing skills of teachers, both special and mainstream, are often inadequate, and so on. For most deaf children there is a stark choice between attending the local school or staying at home, as only a minority can attend any special schools that may exist.

Managua, Nicaragua

In January 2005 Leonard Cheshire Latin America organised a conference on Nicaraguan Sign Language which was attended by 200 deaf children, adults and their families. This was the first time that members of Nicaragua's deaf community had come together to report their experiences to sign language researchers from Nicaragua and the US (LC, 2005). The Nicaraguan deaf community and its achievements in developing an indigenous sign language has received wide international attention.

This example from Nicaragua indicates how much work has to take place in developing a sign language before it can be used to promote educational inclusion. And many deaf people state a preference for segregated education where they can be educated in their first language.

Key challenges

- How can specialist teachers, where they exist, work more closely with mainstream schools?
- How can special schools be transformed into resource centres, where so few resources exist, for the benefit of all disabled children?

REFERENCES

Centre for Studies in Inclusive Education, 2004. *Inclusive education: disabled persons and education in the new UN Disability Convention.* www.csie.org.uk accessed 4/8/04

Department for International Development, 2000. *Disability, Poverty and Development.* London: DFID

Department of Education and Science, 1978. *Special educational needs: report of the Committee of Enquiry into the Education of Handicapped Children and Young People.* Chairman: H.M. Warnock. London: HMSO.

Disability Awareness in Action, 2003. *Disabled Children in Nepal.* London: DAA

Dyson, A., 2004. Inclusive education: a global agenda? In *Japanese Journal of Special Education.* 41 (6), pp 613-625

International Council for the Education of the Visually Impaired, 2003. *The Educator,* Vol. XVI, 1. Birmingham: ICEVI. Available from: www.icevi.org

Inclusion International, 2004. *Millennium Development Goals.* Available from: www.disabilityworld.org/11-12_03/news/unmdg.sthml – accessed 12.07.04

Kaplan, I., 2005. Visualising Inclusion. *Enabling Education,* Issue 9. Manchester: EENET

Leonard Cheshire, 2004. Open Day at School. *Compass,* Issue 20, June-August 2004, pp10-12. London: Leonard Cheshire.

Leonard Cheshire, 2005. Simply Unique. *Compass,* Issue 23, March-May 2005, p11. London: Leonard Cheshire.

Leonard Cheshire, 2005. From Few to Many. *Compass,* Issue 24, June-September 2005, p17. London: Leonard Cheshire.

Miles, S. et al., 2003. *Learning from Difference.* Final Report to DFID. Manchester: EENET

Ogot, O., 2004. *Developing Inclusive Environments.* In Enabling Education, Issue 8. Manchester: EENET

Save the Children UK, 2002. *Schools for All: Including disabled children in education.* London: Save the Children UK

Tomasevski, K., 2004. Are we moving towards all-inclusive education or away from it? Keynote address delivered at Centre for Studies of Inclusive Education conference *"Developing inclusive education: Supporting human rights in mainstream schools." May 2004.* Bristol: Centre for Studies in Inclusive Education

UNESCO, 1994. *Salamanca Statement and Framework for Action.* Paris: UNESCO.

UNESCO, 2001a. *Open File on Inclusive Education: Support Materials for Managers and Administrators.* Paris: UNESCO

UNESCO, 2001b. *Inclusion in Education: The participation of disabled learners.* World Education Forum, EFA 2000 Assessment: Thematic Study. Paris: UNESCO.

UNESCO, 2004. *An inclusive approach to EFA: UNESCO's role.* In Enabling Education, Issue 8, pp 12-13, June 2004. Manchester: EENET.

APPENDIX I: THE KISUMU STATEMENT ON INCLUSIVE EDUCATION – KENYA, 2004

We, participants from ten countries in Africa, Pakistan and the UK meeting at Kisumu, Kenya, at a workshop organised by Leonard Cheshire International, from 9th to 12th May 2004 to share experiences in inclusive education within the African region ten years since the Salamanca Conference and four years after the Dakar Framework for Action (2000).

We observed that:

• Many governments in the region embrace the philosophy of inclusive education *in principle*. However there are no explicit policies and guidelines on the implementation of inclusive education.
• Within the 12 countries represented in the workshop, the understanding of the concept of inclusive education is inconsistent and largely inadequate.
• Major barriers hindering implementation of inclusive education include lack of economic empowerment and social exclusion.

- Inclusive education is a dynamic process and is influenced by factors such as culture and religion.
- Curricula that support inclusive education exist in few countries.
- The context for implementing inclusive education tends to be charity-oriented rather than rights-based – despite policy and legislative changes.

Since many countries in the African region have endorsed the international agenda for education such as Education for All (EFA), Universal Primary Education (UPE), Millennium Development Goals, Standard Rules and the Rights of the Child, we participants affirm that:

- All children have a right to quality education within an inclusive environment and that this education must be culturally appropriate and enable them to maximise their potential.

- The inclusive education process does not only provide education, but also empowers, and is a foundation for the sustainable development of the entire community.

- The needs of diverse learners such as those with hearing impairments and visual handicaps can be addressed in inclusive education.

- The participation of families and the wider community is an integral part of the inclusive education process as the ultimate goal is to maintain the children in their families and communities.

The participants noted that, although it is a decade since the World Conference on Special Needs Education was held in Salamanca, there are still fundamental issues to be addressed if inclusive education is to be realised.

The participants therefore call upon governments in Africa to address the following fundamental issues:

- *Awareness and advocacy for inclusive education*
  Understanding of the concept and philosophy of inclusive education among all stakeholders should be enhanced through capacity building and lobbying. Awareness should also include documentation and sharing of information on successful practices. Advocacy activities in each country should include the use of mass media and also target crucial audiences such as the bi- and multi lateral agencies.

- *Participation of people with special educational needs*
  Policies should be formulated and inclusive education implemented in collaboration with people with 'special educational needs'. Their participation at all levels is paramount if meaningful inclusion is to be achieved.

- *Documentation*
  Data regarding the status of special needs education in the individual countries within the region is necessary for effective planning and resource allocation.

- *Policy development*
  Enabling national and regional policies that restructure education systems to accommodate inclusion through the provision and re-allocation of resources, mobilisation of all stakeholders and creating partnership with other organisations.

- *Poverty*
  Economic empowerment is a vital tool for enhancing the participation of communities in inclusive education and inclusion of children from poor families.

- *Accessible physical and social environment*
  School and community environments must be made user-friendly for all learners in order to enable all children to access the learning environment and social services.

- *Delivery of quality education*
  Learning should be child centred and class size should be reduced.

- *Support services*
  Governments must put in place effective support services such as learning materials, assistive devices and relevant human resources both within the school and in the community.

- *War and natural disasters*
  Ensuring the inclusion of those who had been excluded from education due to natural calamities, wars, ethnic clashes and poverty.

- *Rights*
  There should be a move from a charity-oriented to a more rights-based approach to education for all children – including those identified as having 'special educational needs' or disabilities.

- *Community involvement*

  Community based rehabilitation and other community based approaches should be encouraged to ensure support to those children who are out of school and who may require home-based education and support.

- *Assessment and early intervention*

  Assessment and early intervention should be seen as an integral part of the inclusive education process.

- *Monitoring and evaluation*

  Systems should be put in place to examine continuously the progress being made in the implementation of inclusive education.

APPENDIX 2: RATIONALE FOR INCLUSIVE EDUCATION

A. Rationale for inclusive education

UNESCO

The following rationale for moving towards more inclusive schools, based on the Salamanca Statement, is given in the UNESCO Open File:

- There is an *educational justification*; the requirement for inclusive schools to educate all children together means that they have to develop ways of teaching that respond to individual differences and thus benefit all children.

- There is a *social justification*; inclusive schools are able to change attitudes to difference by educating all children together and form the basis for a just and non-discriminatory society.

- There is an *economic justification;* it is likely to be less costly to establish and maintain schools which educate all children together than to set up a complex system of different types of school specialising in different groups of children. If, of course, these inclusive schools offer an effective education to all of their students, then they are also a more cost-effective means of delivering Education for All.

UNESCO, 2001a, p20

Barriers to inclusive education

The Open File recognises the following barriers to inclusive education:

- weak political will,
- insufficient financial resources and the inefficient use of those available,
- the burden of debt,
- inadequate attention to the learning needs of the poor and the excluded,
- a lack of attention to the quality of learning, and
- an absence of commitment to overcoming gender disparities.

UNESCO, 2001a, p.23

B. Definitions of inclusive education

UNESCO
UNESCO plays a leading role internationally in promoting the concept of inclusive education. The following definition demonstrates UNESCO's move towards a broader vision of inclusion, inspired by Salamanca.

"Inclusion is seen as a process of addressing and responding to the diversity of needs of all learners through increasing participation in learning, cultures and communities, and reducing exclusion within and from education". (UNESCO, 2004)

In parallel, however, and in response to concerns that Education for All initiatives do not necessarily include disabled children, UNESCO has worked with international disability-focused organisations to establish an EFA *Flagship* entitled, "The Right to Education for Persons with Disabilities: Towards Inclusion". Its main goal is to ensure that national EFA plans incorporate disabled people. Some of the contradictions inherent in this Flagship initiative are discussed below.

For more information see www.unesco.org

Department for International Development (DFID)
DFID does not have a policy on inclusive education. However in its 'Disability, Poverty and Development' paper, DFID adopted an equal opportunities perspective:

> "Inclusive education in a developing country implies the equal right of all children to the 'educational package', however basic that package may be." (DFID, 2000, p. 12)

Inclusive education is perceived to be part of an inclusive development approach to international work. DFID's central focus is on eliminating poverty and working towards the Millenium Development Goals (MDGs). The statement above implies that DFID would support initiatives which enable disabled childen to access Universal Primary Education and which support them to complete that primary education.

For more information see www.dfid.gov.uk

The Enabling Education Network (EENET)

In carrying out its work, EENET's overall approach to inclusive education is based on the following assumptions:

- All children can learn.
- Inclusive education is a dynamic process which is constantly evolving.
- Differences in children, such as age, gender, ethnicity, language, disability, HIV and TB status, should be acknowledged and respected.
- Education structures, systems and methodologies should be developed to meet the needs of all children.
- Such developments should be seen as part of a wider strategy to promote an inclusive society.
- Progress need not be restricted by large class sizes or a shortage of material resources.

Definition of inclusive education created at the Agra seminar (EENET 1998)

For more information see www.eenet.org.uk

Inclusive Education in the UK
Non-governmental organisations – UK

Centre for Studies in Inclusive Education (CSIE): Index for Inclusion

The Index for Inclusion was developed in the UK through a process of collaborative research in schools led by education practitioners, academics and disabled people. It provides a framework for practitioners to evaluate their schools and communities and to develop plans to make them more inclusive. The Index is published and disseminated by the Centre for Studies in Inclusive Education, which is based in

Bristol. Advice is offered by CSIE on the adaptation of the materials for use in a range of different cultural contexts.

The definition of inclusion developed as part of the Index process (CSIE, 2002) is as follows:

- Valuing all students and staff equally.
- Increasing the participation of students in, and reducing their exclusion from, the cultures, curricula and communities of local schools.
- Restructuring the cultures, policies and practices in schools so that they respond to the diversity of students in the locality.
- Reducing barriers to learning and participation for all students, not only those with impairments or those who are categorised as 'having special educational needs'.
- Learning from attempts to overcome barriers to the access and participation of particular students to make changes for the benefit of students more widely.
- Viewing the difference between students as resources to support learning, rather than as problems to be overcome.
- Acknowledging the right of students to an education in their locality.
- Improving schools for staff as well as for students.
- Emphasising the role of schools in building community and developing values, as well as in increasing achievement.
- Fostering mutually sustaining relationships between schools and communities.
- Recognising that inclusion in education is one aspect of inclusion in society.

For more informaion see www.csie.org.uk

Disability Awareness in Action (DAA)

An example of a narrower approach, focused solely on disabled learners, comes from Disability Awareness in Action, an international lobby group drawing on a human rights perspective:

"When we refer to 'inclusion', we mean the participation of disabled children through the provision of fully accessible information, environments and support. This can include the provision of barrier-free environments, information in alternate media such as Braille or on tape, acknowledgement of sign as a language and the provision of personal assistant support and interpretation" (DAA, 2003).

For more information see: www.daa.org.uk

Government organisations – UK

The following summary of definitions of inclusion by the various departments show how current government understandings have developed beyond a focus on special needs. It is perhaps inevitable, given the complexity of the issue, that there is not one single agreed definition.

Qualifications and Curriculum Authority (QCA)

The Qualifications and Curriculum Authority has developed the following Inclusion Statement in the National Curriculum which reflects an understanding of inclusion as a process of overcoming barriers to learning:

The statutory inclusion statement on providing effective learning opportunities for all pupils outlines how teachers can modify, as necessary, the National Curriculum programmes of study to provide all pupils with relevant and appropriately challenging work at each key stage. It sets out three principles that are essential to developing a more inclusive curriculum:

a. Setting suitable learning challenges
b. Responding to pupils' diverse learning needs
c. Overcoming potential barriers to learning and assessment for individuals and groups of pupils.

It is important to note that the QCA guidance is primarily concerned with strategies for ensuring access to the curriculum.

For more information see: www.nc.uk.net

Office for Standards in Education (OFSTED)

OFSTED's primary concern is to ensure high standards of education for all pupils. Schools in England are inspected by OFSTED for their performance in relation to the OFSTED definition of 'educational inclusion'. This reflects a broader approach than a focus on children with identified special needs:

•   Educational inclusion is more than a concern about any one group of pupils … It is about equal opportunities for all … It pays particular attention to the provision made for and the achievement of different groups of pupils.

- Pupils with SEN, minority ethnic groups, children "looked after", pupils at risk of exclusion, girls and boys, pupils who need support for English as an Additional Language (EAL), gifted and talented pupils, etc.

For more information see: www.ofsted.gov.uk

The Department for Education and Skills (DfES)

The main concern of the DfES is to ensure that schools comply with the current legal framework with respect to disability and special needs. The DfES issued Statutory Guidance on inclusion to all schools that refers to the 'cultures, policies and practices' of schools and again reflects an understanding in terms of overcoming barriers to learning:

- *Inclusion Guidance:*
  "Inclusion is a process by which schools and LEAs develop their cultures, policies and practices to include pupils [and] actively seek to remove barriers to learning ... Mainstream education will not always be right for every child all of the time."

At the same time the most recent government strategy document redefines inclusion to refer to education in special schools as well as mainstream schools:

- *Removing Barriers to Learning:*
  "We want to break down the divide between mainstream and special schools to create a unified system where all schools and their pupils are included within the wider community of schools".

In summary, there are many different aspects to the government's education policy and so the definitions above have different purposes. The QCA guidance is primarily concerned with strategies for ensuring access to the curriculum; OFSTED is primarily concerned with ensuring high levels of outcome for all; and the DfES guidance is concerned mainly with ensuring compliance with the legal framework. Although that framework strengthens the rights to mainstream placement, that right is not absolute and is in any case conditional upon parental wishes. Since some children are difficult for mainstream schools to educate and since some parents want special schooling, special schools are likely to continue to have a future in the UK.

Appendix 3: international agreements

The UN Convention on the Rights of the Child, 1989

* *Article 2: Non-discrimination*
  This is arguably the most important article for making inclusive education a reality as it focuses on 'non-discrimination'. It states clearly that every article applies equally, and without exception, to all children, irrespective of race, colour, sex, disability, birth or other status.

* *Articles 28 and 29: Access to quality education*
  These articles reinforce the right of all children to education – irrespective of impairment and disability – and require that this should be provided on the basis of equality of opportunity.

* *Article 23: Disabled children's rights*
  This article is ambiguous as it suggests that disabled children need 'special care', and so could be interpreted to mean some form of segregated education.

The right of all children to have access to a quality education was further reinforced by three major international conferences and declarations which took place between 1990 and 2000.

* *Jomtien, 1990*
  EFA was launched at the World Conference on Education for All in Jomtien, Thailand in 1990. The conference concluded that educational opportunities were limited, basic education was limited to literacy and numeracy, and certain marginalised groups were excluded from education altogether. An expanded vision was needed to achieve EFA by 2000. The Jomtien Declaration highlighted the need to universalise education and promote equity by ensuring that girls, women and other under-served groups gain access to education.

* *Salamanca, 1994*
  The World Conference on Special Needs Education was held in Salamanca in 1994 between the conferences in Jomtien and Dakar. Its main aim was to further the objective of Education for All (EFA). "The Salamanca Statement on Principles, Policy and Practice in Special Needs Education" (UNESCO, 1994) provides a framework and guidance on developing inclusive education internationally.

- *Dakar, 2000*

  In 2000 the World Education Forum was held in Dakar to review progress and set new international targets for achieving EFA. The Forum declared that EFA must take account of the needs of a range of marginalised groups, including the poor and the disadvantaged and those with special learning needs.

APPENDIX 4: TRAINING PACKS

There are many inclusive education training packs available which can be used both in teacher education and more widely with education stakeholders in general. Ideally training packs should be developed in the context in which they are used, using local examples, rather than being imported from a very different context. Many locally developed training packs have, however, drawn upon training materials available internationally.

'Special Needs in the Classroom' Teacher Education Resource Pack

This UNESCO Pack was developed by a team of practitioners from all major regions of the world in the early 1990s under the leadership of Professor Mel Ainscow, and first published in 1993. It has been used in over 50 countries and continues to have an impact. Ideally it is used by key facilitators who have had some training in how to make the best use of the Pack. Some practitioners have found it difficult to adapt the Pack to their context, and instead have used some of the ideas in the Pack to create their own training materials. The Pack has recently been revised and is available from UNESCO.

'Index for Inclusion'

The Index, as it is commonly referred to, was developed in the UK by a team of researchers and practitioners, including disabled people. It is a practical guide which helps schools as they go through the process of inclusive school development. It has been translated into many different languages and adapted for use in a wide range of contexts. The experiences of practitioners around the world are currently being compiled into a book for the benefit of others who may wish to use the Index.

'Open File'

UNESCO's Open File contains a set of support materials for managers and administrators where a policy commitment to the principle of inclusive education has been made, or where there is an informal commitment at community level to promote more inclusive practices in education. The Open File suggests how a commitment to inclusion can be nurtured and developed over time so that a fully-functioning inclusive system can emerge.

'Toolkit for Creating Inclusive, Learning-friendly Environments'
The Toolkit was developed by UNESCO Bangkok and published in 2004. It offers a holistic and practical way for schools and classrooms to become more inclusive and gender-sensitive. It is aimed at teachers, school administrators and education planners and contains six detailed booklets on a range of topics. It will be adapted to the needs of specific country contexts and translated into several regional languages.

'Changing Teaching Practices – using curriculum differentiation
to respond to students' diversity'
The purpose of this book is to facilitate and support inclusion in education. It includes suggestions, strategies and learning activities to use in teaching all learners together, no matter what their abilities, disabilities or backgrounds. It was published by UNESCO in 2004 .

In the following examples from Cambodia and Lesotho, inspiration was drawn from international training packs, but the materials have been developed with the local context in mind.

'The Cambodia Pack'
The Disability Action Council of Cambodia is the national coordinating and advisory body on disability and rehabilitation. It plays a key role in promoting inclusive education at national level. In the process of providing on-the-job training to teachers in Cambodian schools, a set of training materials was developed based on individual case studies. These materials were compiled into 'The Cambodia pack' with EENET's help, in 2003. They are now available from EENET's web site, or in CD-ROM format. The Cambodian programme is progressing well despite the overall context of extreme poverty and very high rates of disability because of war and ongoing landmine injuries. It has been involved in training large numbers of teachers.

'Preparing Teachers for Inclusion', Lesotho
This video-based training pack was developed in 1996 in Lesotho by the Ministry of Education's Special Education Unit in collaboration with Save the Children UK. The pack is available from EENET and the manual can be downloaded from EENET's web site. Although the pack is now quite old, it is still in great demand as it shows African teachers implementing inclusive education in overcrowded classrooms in remote rural areas with very few material resources.

CHAPTER 4

ECONOMIC EMPOWERMENT

PETER COLERIDGE

I. INTRODUCTION

PURPOSE

This paper addresses economic empowerment of disabled people, one of four thematic areas in which Leonard Cheshire International focuses its efforts within the field of disability and development. Its purpose is to reflect the current thinking and debates in the area of economic empowerment of disabled people, including outlining different approaches within the field.

ISSUES ADDRESSED

This paper deals with economic empowerment in the broadest sense. It considers key issues in disability, poverty and development, including disability as a rights issue. It outlines international initiatives, which address disability and poverty, and then examines what is meant by empowerment. It goes on to address the economic and social context, access to training, access to capital, access to jobs in the formal economy and the importance of support structures.

SOURCES

The paper is based largely on findings from a research project being conducted for the ILO by the consultant on good practice in community approaches to skills development and access to work for disabled people. The fieldwork for this research was conducted during 2004-5 in Africa (Malawi, Zimbabwe, Uganda and South

Africa), the Middle East (Lebanon and Jordan) and Asia (India, Cambodia and the Philippines).

KEY WORDS

Economic empowerment: the whole subject of vocational skills acquisition, access to work, and employment.

Vocational skills: skills which enhance a person's employability and lift his or her standard of living. These include life skills, interpersonal skills, financial skills, entrepreneurial skills, community skills and technical skills.

Lifelong learning: encompasses all learning activities undertaken throughout life for the development of competencies.

Competencies: denotes the knowledge, skills, attitudes and know-how applied and mastered in a specific context.

Mainstreaming: the process by which disabled people are included as a matter of right in regular services and development programmes provided both by governments and by non-disability-specific organisations.

2. DISABLED PEOPLE AND POVERTY

"We are poor, but we manage. We have enough because we work together. We share. We help each other. We have learned a lot by working together. We have shown that you do not need to depend on outside help. We work in a very simple way, but it is effective. Our children are the ones who benefit in the end." Member of parents' group, USDC CBR programme, Uganda

POVERTY FACTORS

People are poor largely because of external factors outside their control. Conflict, low economic growth, a narrow industrial base, high inflation, low levels of tax collection, low government expenditure, poor standards of healthcare, education, and infrastructure, and rampant corruption, all combine to drive a vicious circle of poverty from which it is extremely difficult for poor individuals to escape.

Disabled people in developing countries tend to be concentrated in the poorest sections of society and it is impossible to separate the poverty of disabled people from this general picture of poverty. On top of all this, disability impoverishes further. Disabled people find it harder to get educated, to access training, and to find employment. If they do find work, it tends to be at a lower level than their true abilities, and they tend to be regarded as expendable in downsizing. If an adult becomes disabled, official safety nets are often non-existent and the affected person and his or her family may slide into a downward spiral of increasing poverty.

So in developing countries poverty is both a cause and a result of disability. It is therefore important for organisations working with disabled people to have a grasp of the factors driving poverty in general. Disability needs to be seen as part of the total picture of poverty affecting developing countries. Most importantly, the cost of disabled people not being economically active needs to be taken into account. If they do not contribute to a family's income, they are considered an economic burden both on the family and ultimately on the state by increasing the general level of poverty.

THE COMPLEX RELATIONSHIP BETWEEN DISABILITY, STATISTICS AND POVERTY

However, the statistical relationship between poverty and disability is complex. What constitutes a disability is to some extent culturally determined, and this makes global comparisons and estimates unreliable. The profile of disability is different between rich and poor countries. In poor countries malnutrition, infectious diseases, war, dangerous work conditions, and lack of medical services especially around birth and trauma, are all poverty related and all cause disability.

The health profile in rich countries is very different and the causes of disability are different. Most significantly, survival rates between rich and poor countries contrast dramatically. Better medical services in rich countries mean that babies born with disabilities such as spina bifida survive. If a person is spinally injured in a car crash in Britain, good medical provision means that the chances of survival for a normal lifespan are high. In a poor country like Malawi the chances of surviving spinal injury for more than a few months are very low. In rich countries partial disabilities associated with old age such as arthritis, hearing loss and reduced vision are common disabling factors.

So, ironically better healthcare and a wealthier lifestyle do not mean less disabled people; they simply change the profile of disabling conditions. Furthermore, low survival rates in poor countries mean that disabled people form a much lower proportion of the population than they do in rich countries. The figure of 10% once used by World Health Organisation (WHO) as a world average is seldom reflected in poor countries, which typically have prevalence figures of less than 5%, with 1-2% being common. The *incidence*[8] figures are generally unknown, but if they were known we would have some idea of how many disabled people die prematurely. Rich countries typically have prevalence figures above 10%. These higher figures are the result of higher survival rates, plus the fact that the state provides incapacity benefits not only to people with physical, sensory and mental impairments, but also to people with conditions which would not be considered disabilities in poor countries, such as chronic depression.

Some organisations working in the disability field, especially DPOs, are reluctant to accept low prevalence figures of disability in poor countries, arguing that they are under-estimates. But the multitude of CBR programmes in developing countries, which have an interest in identifying clients and which work mainly among poor people, provide detailed and very specific local evidence that the low figures are real.[9] It must be understood that *these figures are in themselves a major part of the problem of disability:* they are an indicator of poor health services, low survival rates, lack of awareness and neglect. Low prevalence rates are therefore not a reason for complacency, but are a cause for serious concern. There is little doubt that the low prevalence figures are an important contributory factor in the marginalisation of disabled people. For example, governments in poor countries feel they can ignore disabled people because they do not constitute a significant block of voters.

---

[8] *Incidence* refers to the gross number born disabled or who become disabled.
   Prevalence refers to the net figure of those who survive.

[9] For example, a national CBR programme under UNDP in Afghanistan, a country severely affected by landmines, never found more than 3% in local, house-to-house surveys; it was usually less. Most NGOs working in disability in India use a figure of 2%.

[10] UNESCO figures.

DISABILITY IMPOVERISHES ESPECIALLY
WOMEN AND CHILDREN

Poverty is not simply lack of income; it is a denial of the fundamental freedom and opportunity to develop as a human being. With severely reduced access to education, training, and employment, disabled people face impoverishment in every sense of the word.

Women and children are further marginalised within this scenario. Eighty-seven percent of the world's disabled children live in a developing country, but only 1-2% of them attend any type of formal education[10]. Mortality for disabled children before their fifth birthday may be as high as 80% in some countries.

Disability impacts especially severely on women. The presence of a disabled person in a family affects the whole family, but especially the mother and sisters. Disability may affect not only the marriage prospects of the disabled person, but also those of their siblings through an assumption that the disability is genetic. At the same time, disabled children and women may be victims of sexual abuse. Female genital mutilation and childbirth with inadequate health care may cause disability in women. Furthermore, the burden of care for a disabled family member usually falls on women, increasing the poverty trap by reducing their chances of economic activity, if it is an adult and of education if it is a girl.

The relationship between poverty and disability is discussed further in Section 6, The Importance of the Social and Economic Context.

SUMMARY

1. Disability needs to be seen as part of the overall picture of poverty in developing countries.

2. The profile of disability is different between poor and rich countries. Survival rates in poor countries are very low. Low prevalence rates in poor countries are an important factor in the marginalisation of disabled people.

3. Women and children are especially affected by disability in the family.

3. INTERNATIONAL INITIATIVES TO COMBAT POVERTY RELEVANT TO DISABLED PEOPLE

"The destiny of human rights is in the hands of all our citizens in all our communities."
Eleanor Roosevelt

FRAMEWORKS TO REDUCE POVERTY

There are a number of key global initiatives, which set out a framework for action to reduce poverty. Of particular relevance to this paper are:

- *The Millennium Development Goals (MDGs)*, formulated by the UN in 2000.
- *The Poverty Reduction Strategy Paper (PRSP)* approach.
- *The Global Partnership for Disability and Development*, formulated by the World Bank and other international agencies in 2004. This is the most important international framework for the realisation of the MDGs for disabled people.

The Millennium Development Goals have the following aims:

1. Eradicate extreme poverty and hunger.
2. Achieve universal primary education.
3. Promote gender equality and empower women.
4. Reduce child mortality.
5. Improve maternal health.
6. Combat HIV/AIDS, malaria and other diseases.
7. Ensure environmental sustainability.
8. Develop a global partnership for development.

If they are to be realised, the MDGs need detailed, well-planned, participatory programmes. They cannot be achieved if some people are excluded, including and especially disabled people, for whom all of these aims are directly relevant.

A major mechanism for reaching these goals is the *Poverty Reduction Strategy Paper (PRSP)* approach, adopted by the World Bank in 1999, and now a feature of the planning processes in many developing countries. This approach is designed to create a process of participatory planning within countries, in contrast to the top-down, externally imposed planning of Structural Adjustment policies used by the IMF in the eighties and early nineties, which are seen to have created as many problems as they tried to solve (Coleridge 2006).

The hallmark of the PRSP approach is indeed participation by all stakeholders, including and especially poor people themselves. Participation of the poor is sought at all stages of the PRSP process: formulation, implementation, monitoring and evaluation. However, to date disabled people have found it difficult to make their voices heard in the PRSP process. It is clear that specific initiatives designed to enable them to be heard are required.

GLOBAL PARTNERSHIP FOR DISABILITY AND DEVELOPMENT

The World Bank and other international agencies formulated the Global Partnership for Disability and Development (GPDD) in 2004 in order to provide a framework for disabled people to be included in anti-poverty strategies. The overall objective of the GPDD is to

'Combat the social and economic exclusion and impoverishment of people with disabilities and their families in developing countries by increasing awareness and understanding, and strengthening cooperation among developing country governments, bilateral and multilateral donors, development banks, UN agencies, development NGOs, disabled persons' organisations, NGOs working in the field of disability, foundations, enterprises, and other partners, internationally and nationally' (World Bank 2004).

The GPDD identifies roles for each of the sectors listed in the above objective. The role of international and national NGOs working in the field of disability (of which LCI is one) "will work to assist other partners as well as governments in the formulation of policies and the implementation of programmes to ensure the inclusion of disability issues and the participation of people with disabilities (World Bank 2004).

The design of the GPDD has been determined by six tenets:

a) Use existing administrative structures.
b) Practice both 'parallelism' and 'pooling'.
c) Provide a strong voice for disabled people.
d) Provide for influence from and of developing countries.
e) Think globally, act locally.
f) Complement human rights declarations and conventions.

The GPDD intends to work through two key mechanisms: first, an informal alliance of many stakeholders with the World Bank acting as a secretariat and second, a multi-donor trust fund.

The GPDD implicitly embraces a twin-track approach, in which both mainstreaming and special focus programmes are implemented to secure the rights of disabled people.

ILO CONVENTIONS AND RECOMMENDATIONS

There are in addition a number of ILO Conventions and Recommendations on vocational rehabilitation and employment of disabled people. *Convention 159* (1983) calls upon states to formulate, implement and periodically review a national policy on vocational rehabilitation and employment of disabled people, based on the principles of equal opportunity and equal treatment, aimed at mainstreaming opportunities and services where possible. Measures to be introduced should include vocational guidance, vocational training, placement, employment and other related services, using existing services. The convention had been ratified by 73 states up to 2003 (ILO 2003).

The ILO Code of Practice *'Managing Disability in the Workplace'* (2001) provides guidance on managing disability issues in recruitment, promotion, job retention and return to work. Whereas Convention 159 is aimed at national governments, this Code of Practice is aimed at employers, trade unions, NGOs and DPOs.

The most recent ILO instrument is *Recommendation 195 (2004) Concerning Human Resources Development: Education, Training and Lifelong Learning.* It notes "quality education, pre-employment training and learning throughout life are the three pillars for building and maintaining an individual's employability."

The recommendation is built on a number of core principles that reflect the ILO's values:

- That education, training and lifelong learning contribute significantly to promoting the interests of people, enterprises, the economy and society as a whole.

- That lifelong learning contributes to personal development, access to culture, and active citizenship.

- That many developing countries should be assisted to design, fund and implement education and training policies for economic and employment growth, and the eradication of poverty.

- That education and training are a right for all people. Policies that ensure people with special needs access to education, training and lifelong learning will be a powerful tool to liberate them economically and socially.

SUMMARY

These initiatives and instruments emphasise that:

1. Combating poverty requires a multi-sectoral and multi-actor approach.

2. Combating poverty must be consultative and involve poor people themselves in planning and implementation.

3. The involvement of disabled people in planning and implementation cannot be left to goodwill: it must be strategised.

4. A two-track approach is necessary in which both mainstreaming and special focus programmes are implemented to secure the rights of disabled people.

5. Lifelong learning programmes for personal development need to be available to everyone, including and especially disabled people.

4. DISABILITY AS A RIGHTS ISSUE

"It is quite obvious that 'equal opportunity' and 'equal protection' can only be between those who are equally situated. It is also obvious that treating unequals as equals will result in injustice." Barbara Harriss-White (1995)

THE BASICS

The inclusion of disabled people in economic activity depends to a large extent on the way they are viewed within society and by policy makers. There have been encouraging shifts since the International Decade of Disabled Persons (1981-91) in the way disability is viewed. These shifts can be characterised as follows (ILO 2002):

- Policy and programmes in favour of disabled persons should no longer be viewed as a means to rehabilitate and adapt the disabled individual to society, but to *adapt society to the needs of the disabled individual.*
- The concept of rehabilitation should give way to the concept of *creating an enabling environment.*
- The concept of social assistance should be replaced by one of respect for the *rights of a society's* minorities.
- The minority concept should be embedded into the more inclusive one of *social diversity,* of a *society for all.*

In other words, there has been a revolutionary shift in thinking from the individual medical model, in which the disabled person is required to fit in with the norms of an able-bodied society, to a rights approach based on the social model, in which disabled people have the same rights as anybody else and society must adapt to the needs and rights of disabled people.

However, even though this revolution has occurred among those relating directly to disability, it has not always been understood, let alone embraced, by mainstream planners. As recently as 1993 the United Nations Development Programme (UNDP) Human Development Report made no mention of disabled people whatsoever. And as recently as 2001 the World Bank was still referring to disabled people as *'not able to be economically active, in need of special care and welfare'* in its Sourcebook to the PRSP process (Klugman 2001). And while pro-disability laws have been introduced by many governments in developing countries, the picture is patchy, and implementation almost universally weak.

Strategies need to be put in place to ensure that the shifts described above become a reality on the ground.

CHALLENGES OF THE RIGHTS BASED APPROACH

The state is the only institution capable of creating and implementing the rights of its citizens. That is its function and purpose. NGOs can lobby, but they cannot enact laws. But hard-pressed, cash-strapped governments generally speaking are reactive; they grease the squeaky wheel. Priorities are determined by what will win votes, or at least by what will reduce opposition. Because disabled people are not perceived to constitute a block of sufficient size to influence elections (a factor directly related to the low prevalence figures), and because the perceived economic and administrative costs are considered high for little obvious economic return, politicians do not see disability as a priority. It is the task of NGOs and DPOs to make sure that the rights of disabled people are seen as a political as well as a moral priority. This requires time, energy, resources and effective strategies.

Many DPOs and disability-focused NGOs have got this message. Some have diverted their energies to lobbying and away from direct service provision. This is especially so in the field of economic empowerment.

In theory this is admirable; in practice it may mean that disabled people become more marginalised. There are two main reasons for caution.

First, lobbying may work where a government has both cash and commitment (as for example in South Africa), but is not likely to work where the government does not have the means to provide the most basic services to its general population. Reducing an NGO's activities to advocacy for inclusion may mean that disabled people receive no services at all. Furthermore, some advocacy activists have reached the conclusion, after many years of trying, that government systems cannot be reformed (Satish 2001).

Second, advocacy, with all the workshops, seminars and 'capacity building' that accompany it, can easily be cornered by educated middle-class development workers to the exclusion of poor people themselves. In such programmes very few resources reach ordinary people, and disparities within a society increase (Satish 2001).

One of the main advantages of community based service delivery programmes is that they keep those in need clearly in focus, and allow development workers and planners to keep in touch with the reality and aspirations of disabled people.

A TWIN-TRACK APPROACH

Advocacy for mainstreaming alone will not secure the rights of disabled people. Unlike other minority groups, disabled people have particular needs before they reach the starting blocks of equality. 'Treating unequals as equals will only result in injustice.' (Satish 2001).

So an organisation like LCI needs to adopt a twin-track approach in which it both provides direct services and serves as an advocate for inclusion in mainstream services. This approach is of particular importance in economic empowerment, as will be made clear in the rest of this paper.

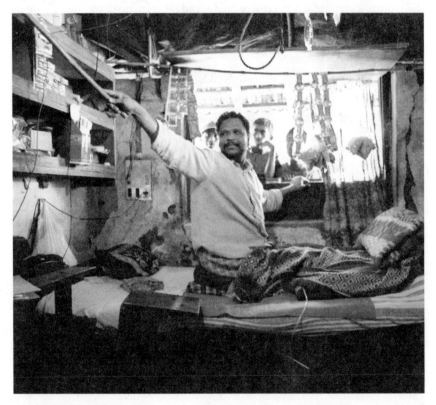

Photo: Mimi Mollica / Leonard Cheshire

Disabled people's organisations have a crucial role to play in the formulation, articulation and monitoring of a rights based approach to disability. There are a number of successful examples around the world where DPOs have been instrumental in persuading their government to adopt better legislation on disability: South Africa, Zimbabwe in the early years after independence, and Lebanon during and after the civil war which ended in 1992 are examples known at first hand by the author, but there are many others. These examples can give encouragement to DPOs everywhere in what is often felt to be an uphill struggle. DPI (Disabled Peoples International) is an important rallying point internationally, although DPI is not always connected to grass roots representation.

However, it is not only at the level of government lobbying that DPOs need to be active. Small, local DPOs at community level can play an important role in the empowerment of disabled people and their families, and can be effective in enabling the voices at grass-roots level to be heard at national level. However, community level DPOs are often unfunded and have considerable communications problems. Agencies such as LCI can encourage such local organisations by ensuring that they are included in local programme planning, implementation and monitoring.

(A fuller treatment of the rights based approach can be found in *Disability and Poverty.'* Leonard Cheshire July 2004.)

SUMMARY

1. The social model of disability has gained currency among disability-focused organisations, but understanding in the mainstream remains weak.

2. The existence of pro-disability laws is not the same as a pro-disability policy and strategy.

3. Advocacy for inclusion in the mainstream is important but on its own is not sufficient to ensure the rights of disabled people.

4. A twin-track approach is needed, combining advocacy with service provision.

5. DPOs have a crucial role in formulating, articulating and monitoring a rights based approach at international, national and community levels.

5. WHAT DOES EMPOWERMENT MEAN?

"If people feel good about themselves, they can start to create change." B. Venkatesh, India

THE VICIOUS CIRCLE OF DISEMPOWERMENT

Disabled people are affected by a negative spiral of factors, which drive them into low expectations, low self-esteem, and low achievement. This spiral is illustrated in the diagram below.[11]

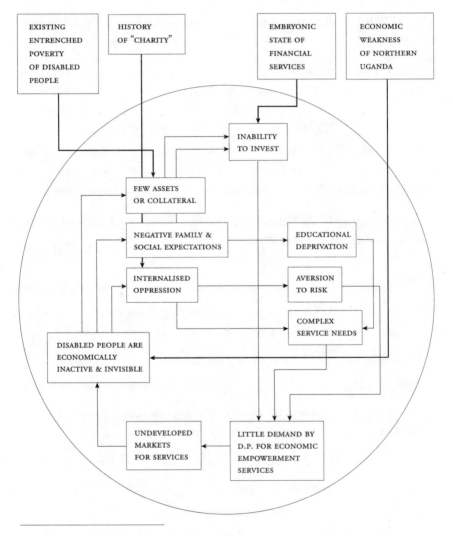

[11] With acknowledgement to Mike Albu: *Improving Business Development Services with Disabled People in Northern Uganda. Evaluation of an action-research project by NUDIPU and APT Enterprise Development.* July 2005.

The main purpose of this paper is to explore ways in which this vicious spiral can be broken.

It is not only a matter of discrimination, it is also a matter of personal empowerment. In research into economic empowerment of disabled people for the ILO undertaken in Africa, the Middle East, and Asia, it was found that the hallmark of a disabled person who is successful in work is that they are outgoing, positive, and *concerned about the well being of others as well as themselves* (Coleridge 2005). This was often seen in the way they made friends with their customers, their involvement in the community through membership of groups or committees, and at times their support of disabled children outside their immediate family. In other words, it was those who were most empowered and self-confident as individuals who were most successful in their business. Conversely, those who were depressed, isolated, and full of complaints were the least successful.

A strategy needs to identify the factors which empower (and also those which disempower) disabled people, and which enable them to live more productive lives, with greater self-esteem and respect from their community.

EMPOWERMENT ILLUSTRATED BY ONE CASE STUDY

One case study from Uganda illustrates the point: development worker and vet David Luyombo, who became disabled by polio at the age of three.

David attended primary school largely because his mother insisted that he did so. His father was not interested in him, because of his disability. The school was four miles away, and he had to walk. (He walks with some difficulty with a stick.) After completing primary school, he attended a boarding secondary school in Kampala and then went to a tutorial college where he got a diploma in bookkeeping and secretarial work.

But he was strongly motivated to work for the development of disabled people in his home rural area in Masaka, and did not see working as an accounts clerk in Kampala as a way to achieve that aim.

David says: *"I wanted to say no to my own experience of limited opportunities, stereotyping and discrimination. I wanted to prove that real development with disabled people in rural areas in Uganda is possible. Traditionally, disabled people, if they are taught anything at all, are taught handicrafts, which are very difficult to sell in rural areas. It seemed to me that the only thing that made sense was farming, and in particular livestock."*

So he trained as a veterinary technician on a distance-learning course at Makere University.

On qualifying in 1990 he became a self-employed vet technician in Masaka. Neither donor agencies nor NUDIPU (the principle Ugandan DPO) believed that there was much scope for employment opportunities for disabled people in rural areas.

David began to breed good quality cows, goats, pigs, turkeys and chickens, and to train disabled people and their families in better animal husbandry. He gave animals to families with a disabled member on condition that they gave him the first offspring, which could then be given to another family.

Despite the fact that polio made it hard for him to use a bicycle, he cycled all over the rural areas of his home district to identify families with disabled people. He focused on families, and not simply on individuals, for two reasons: first, in some cases the disabled person was a child and not ready to earn an income, or unable to do so due to severe impairments. Second, involving the whole family enabled them to see the disabled person as an asset, not as a liability.

By the end of 1990 he had 13 members in the association he was forming. Today there are over 500. Each member pays a small membership fee, which is the main source of income for the association as an organisation. It was slow at the start because people did not think he was serious, and did not want to make a financial commitment to something that, they thought, had little future. But when he reached 50 members people began to realise he was serious. He was able to acquire a small motorbike, which made his access to families quicker and easier.

David realised early on that to train people in better animal husbandry required a model farm and a training centre with accommodation, where people could come for training courses lasting several days. This is what he is in the process of building. The model farm is there, with Friesian cows, crossbred goats and pigs, and good quality turkeys and chickens kept in well-constructed pens. The accommodation is already built and the training centre itself is almost completed.

The training centre could become a resource for rural development in the whole of Uganda.

The qualities that characterise David are clear:

- He has a large vision, but started small.

- He identified the most obvious source of income for rural farming families: livestock, not crafts.
- He works with families, not with individuals.
- He works by demonstration.
- He has linked disability to other development issues.
- He has attracted the notice of people in mainstream development who have never linked their work with disabled people.

David's sense of empowerment is reflected in his ambition to help others rather than just himself. He is making a success of his life because of a driving aspiration for development – of people, of disabled people, and of his area. This leads him to think creatively and positively, to plan, to continually seek ways to improve what he finds. He has become one of the driving forces for the development of a wider rural community.

David is an empowered individual, a powerful role model who provides a focus of aspiration for other disabled people.

As David illustrates, success is dependent not so much on technical skills (though he has those) but on core life skills, attitudes, and knowledge. These include interpersonal skills, financial skills, entrepreneurial skills, and community skills, as well as technical skills. The key concept is 'value added': what skills are needed to add value to a person's life to make them more able to engage in work that is fulfilling and enables them to earn a decent wage? This question is treated below in Section 7, Access to Training.

SUMMARY

1. Disabled people start with a major disadvantage in the employment stakes: negative attitudes in society and low self-esteem.
2. Economic empowerment programmes need to find strategies for breaking out of this vicious circle.
3. Disabled people who are most successful in economic activities are those who are concerned for, and work towards, the well-being of others as well as themselves.
4. Role models of such disabled people are the most valuable way of demonstrating how the vicious circle can be broken. Role models provide examples of both hope and aspirations for other disabled people.

6. THE IMPORTANCE OF ECONOMIC AND SOCIAL CONTEXT

> "Development work is primarily about three things: awareness, awareness, and awareness." Renaldo Retief, Kenya

THE STRATEGY MUST BE MATCHED TO THE CONTEXT

Without an awareness of the wide range of social, economic and legislative contexts in developing countries, discussion of development issues becomes unreal. Consider the following table:[12]

Country	Gross National Income Per capita	Life expectancy	Infant mortality
Malawi	$160	37	113/1000
South Africa	$2,780	46.5	52/1000
Lebanon	$4,040	71	28/1000

These figures illustrate a wide range of economic and development contexts. Lebanon has a GNI (Gross National Income measured per capita) 25 times that of Malawi, a life expectancy which is double, and an infant mortality rate one quarter of Malawi's.

The social and legislative context in relation to disabled people also differs widely between countries. This may or may not be in parallel with the general level of education, which is linked to the economy. Uganda, with much lower levels of education than Lebanon, is the only country in the world where the representation of disabled people at all levels of government from village council to parliament is constitutionally required.[13] By contrast, until the end of the civil war in Lebanon in 1992, it was against the law for the government to employ disabled people as civil servants. This has now been changed as a result of work done by DPOs in Lebanon since the end of the war.

---

[12] World Bank figures 2003.

[13] This extraordinary achievement is largely the result of effective lobbying by NUDIPU (National Union of Disabled People of Uganda)

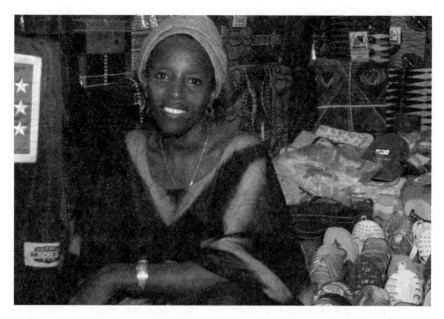

These enormous economic, social and political differences between countries pose a significant challenge to any attempt to provide general guidelines on development issues, in particular in the field of economic empowerment. Whatever the reasons for these enormous differences, an economic empowerment programme must be based on the local reality and not on some theoretical concept.

FORMAL VERSUS INFORMAL ECONOMY

The most obvious difference between countries like Lebanon and Malawi is the size of the informal versus the formal economy. In many African countries, up to 80% of the workforce is engaged in the informal economy, in India it is 93%. This will rise with increasing globalisation and deregulation of the international market, as well as population increases, which outstrip economic development.

The informal economy is unregulated in the sense that people who work in it generally do not pay direct taxes, and have no state pensions or other benefits. It is regarded with ambivalence by governments: on the one hand it does not contribute to the national exchequer by paying direct taxes, and includes illegal or shadowy activities such as prostitution and local alcohol production. On the other hand it provides jobs for millions of people, and contributes a substantial percentage of the GDP (e.g. Uganda 20%, Kenya 30%) (Haan no date).

In terms of training and preparation for work, it is essential to bear in mind the substantial differences between work in the formal and informal economies. The following table summarises the main differences:

FORMAL ECONOMY	INFORMAL ECONOMY
– Usually governed by employment law (which may be pro-disability)	– Unregulated and therefore employment law not applied
– Provides a job with a regular salary and benefits	– Income may be derived from several activities either individually or as part of a family unit. Concept of a 'job' not necessarily applicable
– Very few formal jobs in rural areas. Most formal jobs require urban residence	
– Good level of education and literacy required (usually minimum of secondary)	– In rural areas informal is usually the only option. Being a contributor to family and community may be more important than a job
– Technical skills needed, including administrative skills. Entrepreneurial skills not usually required except by owners or managers.	– Literacy and numeracy important but secondary level of education not essential – can be seen as a disadvantage if it leads to unfulfilled expectations
– Core life skills essential	– Entrepreneurial skills essential
– Ability to work within an organisation, system or structure. Strong initiative not essential	– Core life skills essential
– Individual does not require capital	– Ability to be self-initiating and independent is vital. Good networking and community skills needed
– Savings important but not vital to work success	
– Support derived from employment structure and colleagues	– Requires capital. Basic financial skills essential
	– Ability to save essential if business is to prosper
	– Support derived from savings and community groups

Clearly, preparing people for work in the formal economy is very different from preparation for the informal economy.

The informal economy provides the most likely opportunities for work for disabled people in poor countries.

Much has been written on the informal economy, but because it covers such a wide range of activities agreement on its definition remains elusive. However, it is helpful to distinguish three broad types of activity within it (Haan no date):

a) *Income-generating activities (IGAs):* usually rural subsistence-type self-employment often supplementing another form of income such as farming with women as the dominant actors. Typically part-time, seasonal activities based on traditional technologies, local materials and local markets. They have little if any potential for growth and might be best supported by assisting women to diversify their activities e.g. seasonal trading and hawking, pig and poultry raising, traditional crafts.

b) *Micro-enterprises (MEs):* larger than IGAs, they constitute the principle source of income for those engaged in them. MEs may involve an entire family or a group of families, and may have employees. They may be involved in providing a service or in production for a local market, have modest technical skills and no management to speak of e.g. small shops, metalworking, carpentry, tailoring, repair services.

c) *Small enterprises (SEs):* employ workers (up to 50). May use 'modern' (non-traditional) technologies. Their services and products range from simple to complex. SEs are on the margins of the formal economy and may pay some taxes. Usually urban based e.g. saw mills, garment assembly, construction, medium-scale agro-processing.

The main differences between these three are summarised in the table below:

IGAs	MEs	SEs
Mixed with household economy	Mixed with household economy but shifting towards separation	Separate from household economy
Self-employment (with some help from family members)	Up to 10 workers, mostly family members + apprentices	10 – 50 employees
Few or no fixed assets (less than $500)	Moderate fixed assets (less than $10,000)	Fixed assets up to $100,000
Traditional, manual technologies	Mixed but obsolete technologies	More modern technologies
Profits for household consumption	Profits for household consumption and in business	Profits for reinvestment in business
Diversification to increase household income and minimize risk	Specialisation to increase household income	Specialisation to increase profits

The combination of poor education and the high costs of transport often mean that people living in poor circumstances have very limited horizons. They do not have the information they need for proper market research, do not have views of good examples, and do not have the tools for analysis to lead them to a better future. With their greater mobility problems this is especially true for disabled people.

A major problem in countries where the informal sector is dominant is that the government's ambivalence may be expressed by heavy-handedness. Instead of providing a legislative and infrastructural context that enhances the chances of small informal businesses being successful, it may actively harass them. In Nairobi, for example, the municipality regularly tears down roadside stalls without providing any alternative site or compensation. In May 2005 the Zimbabwean government arrested more than 9,000 petty traders on the streets of Harare and destroyed their stalls. Local governments may also place enormous bureaucratic impediments in the way of legitimate small businesses, which want to expand.

There is a clear need for organised lobbying to make the informal sector more recognised and appreciated for both the services it provides and the jobs it creates. Disabled people through their organisations need to add their voice to this lobbying process.

THE IMPACT OF GLOBALISATION ON JOBS AND EMPLOYABILITY

Labour market conditions have deteriorated sharply under the impact of globalisation and keen competition. Manufacturing businesses in developing countries are downsizing their workforces, and contracting out to home production units where they have no responsibility for recruitment or the welfare of workers. This is driving increasing numbers into the informal economy, where there are no benefits and where employment law, including quotas and minimum wages, is not enforced. Vulnerable groups – disabled people, young people, women, and older workers – are the primary victims.

On the other hand, despite these very negative trends, globalisation does present positive opportunities hinging on the principle of corporate responsibility, a growing factor with consumer pressure organisations in western countries. This has impacted especially on, for example, child labour, and has forced firms like Nike to look at the conditions in which their outworkers produce footballs in Pakistan. It could also operate in favour of disabled people, if consumers put pressure on multi-nationals to adopt full equal opportunities policies. Some firms like Marks and Spencer have already shown openness to such pressure and have committed themselves to employing disabled women as garment makers in Sri Lanka.

RURAL VERSUS URBAN

Rural areas throw up fundamental questions about development in general and for disabled people in particular. If fulfilling aspirations and improving one's standard of living are what development is about, how far can better aspirations be realised in rural areas which are mainly dependent on small-scale farming? Some disabled people, notably those who are visually impaired, can function better with their brains than with their hands, but the opportunities for personal development for disabled people in rural areas may be limited.

Rural areas are, however, as diverse as any other areas of development, and generalisation are dangerous. One of the former homelands in South Africa, where people live in low-grade housing settlements with little or no access to agricultural land, presents different constraints and opportunities from Uganda, where rural families tend to have land that they can farm.

In rural areas where the economy is based on small-scale agriculture, there are very few 'jobs' in the conventional sense. Therefore the aim in rural areas must be to identify skills and activities that will sustain and enhance the quality of life in a subsistence environment (Murray 1985). The need is to find opportunities for disabled people to make a contribution to family and village-level life, both economically and socially, rather than think in terms of a clearly identified and self-sufficient job. If the family is able to farm, then the best option is to strengthen their income from farming by, for example, training them in better livestock production, rather than training the disabled member in a different skill such as tailoring. In rural areas, especially, a village of say 500 people may have a number of tailors, and training one more will not provide much of an income. Farming provides much better prospects.

David Luyombo, the disabled vet in Uganda quoted earlier, understands this point very well. He said: *"Traditionally, disabled people, if they are taught anything at all, are taught handicrafts, which have a very limited market in rural areas. It seemed to me that the only thing that made sense was farming, and in particular livestock."* He now runs a model farm and training centre in Masaka to teach people better animal husbandry.

FOCUS ON THE WHOLE FAMILY, NOT JUST THE DISABLED PERSON

The presence of a disabled person in a family, whether he or she is the main breadwinner or a child, affects the whole family. Families in poor communities usually have survival strategies involving several sources of income. So any employment support activity must take the whole family into account, and, if possible, involve other members of the family in the training process and access to capital. The idea that the disabled person should be entirely self-sufficient in the sense of not needing any help from others is not necessarily a valid concept: mutual support and cooperation is the key. 'Self-employment' and 'self-sufficiency' are sometimes misleading concepts.

Take for example Enifa Stande, a blind teashop owner in Malawi.

Aged 43, married with two sons, Enifa became blind through glaucoma in 2002 at age 41 after three years of gradually losing her sight. She can still see a little light and shade. At first this made her very depressed but a field worker taught her daily living skills and now she manages well.

Before becoming blind she ran a successful tea shop in a busy trading centre, and continues this now, earning between K2000 and K4000 a week. (A handsome income.) Her husband helps her by getting firewood and supplies. She is building two houses to rent with the proceeds.

She and her husband own three acres on which they grow maize. She wants to grow cotton for cash. She does not work on the land. Her husband and hired casual labour do this.

Attitudes towards her have not changed since she became blind. This was evident in the teashop, where there was a friendly atmosphere and a sense of everybody helping each other.

Enifa says: *"becoming blind two years ago was at first a great blow to me. I fell into a big depression. But my husband and others helped me, and now it does not bother me much. I enjoy my work. There is always a lot going on. This teashop is well placed, and people drop in all the time. What are my goals? I would like to go on building houses for rent and possibly start a grocery shop."*

Socially and economically Enifa's life has not changed much since she went blind two years ago. She and her husband have a good income from the teashop. It is clear that she is a valued and respected member of the community. She is obviously providing a valued service – a place where people can meet and talk. Her husband has been a very important source of help for her. Far from rejecting her, he has supported her and together their life works.

David Luyombo, the vet quoted above, insists that it is the family, not just the disabled person, which must be the target for his programme of distributing animals. This means that even disabled people who would not normally be considered a good subject for an income-generating project, for example a child with cerebral palsy, become an asset for the family, not a liability.

SUMMARY

1. An understanding of the economic, social and legislative context is vital when planning economic empowerment programmes.
2. The vast majority of people in work in developing countries work in the informal economy, which also provides the most opportunity for disabled people.
3. The informal economy requires different qualities in its workforce from the formal.
4. 'Jobs' and 'employment' are not useful concepts in rural areas dependent on subsistence agriculture.
5. Economic empowerment programmes in rural areas need to look for ways in which disabled people can contribute to family income, especially through agriculture.
6. It is essential to include the family in economic empowerment programmes, and not focus only on the disabled person.

7. ACCESS TO TRAINING

"We live by encouragement and die without it. Slowly, sadly, and angrily." Celeste Holm

INTRODUCTION

Like non-disabled people, disabled people need skills for economic empowerment. But unlike non-disabled people they start with a number of disadvantages that need to be addressed in training programmes. Successful training strategies have a holistic, developmental approach, which recognises the importance of personal empowerment, the economic and social context, access to capital, and the wide range of skills, knowledge and attitudes needed to succeed in work.

Traditional vocational training institutions, which focus on teaching technical skills alone, have not, in general, proved successful at getting disabled people into work. Similarly community apprenticeship schemes that focus only on technical skill training have generally not proved successful.

COMPETENCIES

Rather than think in terms of skills alone, it is useful to think of competencies. These include attitudes, knowledge and skills, and are illustrated in the diagram below:

ATTITUDES	KNOWLEDGE	SKILLS
– Self-confidence	– Knowledge of the	– Community skills
– Determination	economic context	– Interpersonal skills
– Having aspirations	– Knowledge of the	– Financial skills
– Social responsibility	social context	– Literacy & numeracy
– Willingness to	– Understanding of	– Goal setting
take risks	job market	– Problem solving
– Optimism	– Understanding of	– Opportunity seeking
– Friendliness	market for products	– Information seeking
– Persistence in the	and services	– Planning and
face of set-backs	– Understanding of	monitoring
– Creativity	disability issues	– Bookkeeping
– Risk taking		– Market analysis
– Openness to		– Technical skills
other views		
– Critical thinking		
– High personal		
standards		

TRAINING IN ENTREPRENEURIAL SKILLS:
AN EXAMPLE FROM SOUTH AFRICA

One training establishment that has understood the need for including these competencies in its training courses is MODE in Soweto, South Africa[14].

Key components and hallmarks of the MODE course are target setting, identification of support networks, critical thinking, openness to other views, recognition that people have different ideas of what constitutes success, problem solving, and

---

[14] Medunsa Organisation for Disabled Entrepreneurs

creativity. They also identify their personal entrepreneurial characteristics under the headings of:

- Opportunity seeking
- Goal setting
- Persistence
- Information seeking
- Commitment to work contract
- Systematic planning and monitoring
- Demand for equality and efficiency
- Persuasion and networking
- Risk taking
- Self confidence

This is preliminary to formulating a business plan and the mechanics of running a business.

Surveys have shown an outstanding survival rate for businesses established after MODE training. The majority of businesses started after MODE training generate about R1500 ($245) a month, which is twice the disability benefit. Some grow to earn R3000 ($490), with the potential for further expansion.

One example: Mpho Motshabi started with one shoe repair business and then expanded to two. He also started making sandals. His shoe repair business had to close after a year because passing trade dropped when the taxi route it was on changed. But he kept the sandal-making going and realised that there was demand for fashionable 'ethnic' sandals made from animal skins (e.g. zebra) with the fur still on. He now makes 40-60 pairs a day, exports to Botswana, Namibia and Swaziland, employs six people, and cannot keep up with demand. His turnover is R40-50,000 a month (over $2,000).

The success of the MODE training can be ascribed to the following factors (among others):

- Commitment by trainees to setting up a business. (If they do not, they have to refund the R1500 grant for the course.)
- Aptitude screening.
- The course focuses on life skills as well as business skills.

- Incremental learning building on existing knowledge and skills.
- Close examination of his/her business idea by each trainee throughout the course.
- Thorough research by MODE among disabled persons to understand their levels of skill and education.
- The opportunity for greatly enhanced self-respect among disabled people.
- A holistic and empowering approach, which builds on people's strengths.

Each course trains 15 people, and there is a long waiting list. The main problem for MODE is how to expand organically without running into the problems of dilution. But it is clearly an approach that needs to be applied much more widely than in one site in Johannesburg. It is an example of an idea that needs to be replicated, but which is also viewed protectively by its authors.

In the rest of this chapter we examine other types of training and consider their advantages and disadvantages.

TRADITIONAL VOCATIONAL TRAINING CENTRES (VTCS)

In the past, segregated vocational training centres teaching such skills as shoe making, tailoring, and carpentry were seen as the best way of giving disabled people employable skills, but these are now recognised as having a number of drawbacks. First, they only offer a limited range of trades, and tend to be inflexible in response to a changing market. Second, many of those trained do not get employment, at any rate not in the trade they had been trained in. Third, many disabled people do not want to be limited to these fairly menial types of work, but to have opportunities which are intellectually more challenging. Blind people in particular can benefit from employment opportunities that use their brains rather than their hands. Fourth, because the graduates often cannot find work outside, these VTCs tend to become sheltered workshops, disconnected from the real job market. Fifth, and most importantly, traditional VTCs seldom teach the core competencies listed above.

Alternative forms of training are required, which are more closely attuned to the reality of the market and which offer many more choices than the limited menu of a traditional VTC. A number of alternatives are now tried and trusted: apprenticeship training, entrepreneurial training, training disabled people in a mainstream VTC, and turning a traditional VTC into a community resource.

APPRENTICESHIPS

In apprenticeship training a disabled person is paired with a skilled person (either disabled or non-disabled) already in successful self-employment, who provides training on his or her business site either with or without payment. This is ideally suited to the informal economy. The advantages of apprenticeships are:

1. The trainee relates to the general public throughout the training period, gaining valuable experience in life skills, and sensitising the public to the fact that a disabled person can perform like anyone else.
2. The trainee can pick up much about entrepreneurial skills without formal instruction, but by observation and experience.
3. A much wider range of skills can be offered than in a VTC. These are limited only by the range of people prepared to act as trainers.

The main drawbacks of the apprenticeship approach are:

1. Not all skilled trades-people are good trainers, and some may simply use the disabled person as free labour.
2. No official certification is possible.

TRAINING DISABLED PEOPLE IN A MAINSTREAM VTC

There is no reason why people with mobility impairments should not be included in mainstream VTCs, since the only real problem is access. But mainstream VTCs tend to react against training disabled people on the grounds that they think it is too complicated or that they will not succeed.

The answer is for community based disability programmes to build linkages with mainstream VTCs and work for the inclusion of disabled people on a step-by-step, case-by-case basis. Once one or two have been shown to succeed it will be easier to convince such centres to take on disabled people as a matter of principle.

But as the success of MODE shows, careful selection is vital. Not every disabled person has the aptitude for such training.

USING A VTC AS A COMMUNITY RESOURCE:
AN EXAMPLE FROM JORDAN

The Holy Land Institute for the Deaf (HLID) in Jordan provides high quality education for deaf boys and girls from 4-18, and innovative vocational training for both boys and girls. Its vocational training programme has long been a model of its type. The trades it teaches are traditional – carpentry, metal work and motor mechanics for boys; handicrafts, embroidery and rug weaving for girls – but the way they are taught and their relation with outside markets are not. The workshops are designed to face the street, not the school. The car body repair and motor mechanics shops are set up like any other workshop where people can bring their vehicles to be mended. Trainees relate directly to the customers, which has a number of advantages: it means that the customers get used to dealing with deaf people and the trainees learn how to deal with customers and the realities of the market at first hand. These workshops have established a reputation for quality and now draw customers from well beyond the town where they are sited.

HLID demonstrates that it is possible to combine skills training with production for sale. The carpentry and metal workshops produce for a carefully studied market. For example, in a country with probably more sheep than people, there is a demand for durable sheep handling equipment for dipping, weighing, vaccinating etc. These workshops have designed and make such equipment. They also have a contract to make school furniture, and regularly take orders from embassies for high quality office furniture.

The sewing, embroidery and rug weaving is traditional Palestinian and desert Bedouin, which appeals to tourists. The school has recently established a sales outlet for some of its products in the Jordan Valley beside the Dead Sea (a major tourist area). The building has been designed to use minimum electricity (no air conditioners) and to use natural cooling systems on the principle of air drafts flowing over water. This is another example of the creativity that characterises the school, and is also a demonstration that such a school does not have to limit its focus to disability.

The school has identified tourism as a key target area for both its products and its graduates. The hotel industry is an area that can employ deaf people as cooks, maintenance workers, electricians, and other workers. An ex-hotelier now works as a volunteer with the school, identifying niches where graduates from the school can be placed.

In these and other ways the school is acting as a key community resource.

LIFELONG LEARNING

Increasingly in discussions about education and vocational training generally (not specifically related to disability) the concept of one-shot training courses is being modified by a realisation of the importance of lifelong learning. It is not possible to teach all the attitudes, knowledge and skills needed to succeed in work in one course lasting a few weeks or months. Acquiring the competencies listed above is a cumulative process lasting a lifetime. People learn in different ways, and are ready for some learning at certain times in their lives and not at others. They learn through directed training, by observation of others, by encouragement of friends and family, by their own experience, by testing things out, by failing and trying again.

Any training programme needs to recognise the need for lifelong learning, and build in ways of dealing with it. In particular the need for support and encouragement once the training course is over is paramount. This is treated in more detail in Section 10, The Importance of Support Structures.

SUMMARY

1. Skills are vital for access to work, but must be interpreted more widely than technical skills alone.

2. Competencies include attitudes, knowledge and skills, all of which need to figure in training.

3. An example from South Africa illustrates the success of well-conceived entrepreneurial training that incorporates attitudes, knowledge and skills.

4. The advantages and disadvantages of traditional VTCs, community apprenticeship schemes and mainstreaming are given.

5. Lifelong learning must be built into any training strategy.

8. ACCESS TO CAPITAL

"No capital, no self-employment." Moses Kijongo, Uganda

INTRODUCTION

Most poor people in developing countries do not have access to salaried, formal employment – indeed that is why they are poor. The majority depend on very modest earnings from either selling their labour (cheaply) or producing goods or services, both in the informal economy.

No amount of training will lead to self-employment in the informal economy unless the trainee has access to start-up capital. Lack of access to capital is the most common reason why trainees from vocational training courses (whether institution based or apprenticeships) do not enter employment. There are two principal methods for accessing capital: through micro-finance, and through savings.

MICRO-FINANCE

Micro-finance is a generic term applying to small loans to poor people who do not have access to regular bank loans because they have no collateral. The concept of making small loans to groups whose members can act as collateral for each other was pioneered in Bangladesh primarily by the Grameen Bank, and has become a major tool for development in some countries in Asia. In Africa it has been slower to catch on but micro-finance institutions (MFIs) are springing up there too.

But generally speaking disabled persons are finding that these bodies will not lend to them because they are seen as a poor risk. In addition, many of these bodies operate a group guaranteed loan scheme, but it is hard for disabled people to be accepted into these groups because non-disabled people do not believe they will be able to repay. It is hard for them to form their own disabled groups because they are often too far apart (another consequence of low prevalence figures), especially in rural areas, and may have limited mobility.

Furthermore, even when they do have access to loans through specially targeted programmes, disabled people have traditionally been recipients of charity, and the idea that they should repay a loan rather than receive a grant frequently meets with resistance. This was a principal finding of an evaluation of an ILO loan scheme targeted at disabled people in Kenya in 1993 (Metts et al. 1993). However, the evaluation of this project, despite identifying serious problems with selection, training, loan approval, follow-up assistance, and repayment, also reported important positive findings. Most notably a majority of loan recipients claimed that their self-confidence and status within their family and community had been enhanced. The loan recipients in this programme were all people who already had a business, which needed an injection of capital to make it more viable, and the majority had succeeded in this aim as a result of the loan.

Access to capital remains the key to the establishment and development of micro-enterprises. In Africa in particular where micro-loans have not been a great success, savings strategies have demonstrated traditional African survival strategies that are also the dominant feature of community development in India.

SAVINGS

If micro-credit is not available, the best option for accessing capital is through savings. Even if micro-credit is an option, savings is still a vital discipline that needs to be built into all loan programmes.

The traditional merry-go-round system
In poor communities all over the world a common type of savings is what is called in Kenya the merry-go-round. Here a group comes together for the sole purpose of saving. Each member puts a fixed sum into a common pot each week or each month, the amount agreed by the group to reflect the realistic possibilities of group members. Each month (or whatever interval is agreed by the group) one person from the group takes a turn in scooping the pot. So, for example, if each member of a group of five puts $3 into the pot each month, every month one person will have $15. This can be used for a peak expenditure such as a school uniform, or for investment in an income generating activity, such as buy-ing extra stock for a shop or materials for a workshop.

A modified version of the merry-go-round
A variation on this system being used extensively in India, for example, is to use the amount scooped from the pot as a loan and not a grant. So the recipient pays

it back, at a rate of interest and over a period agreed by the group. In this way the pot is always growing in size, instead of remaining limited to what is put in each month. Over a period of a year or more a relatively large amount of capital can be saved, which could be used for investment in a piece of machinery or the building of a workshop. Or it could be used as collateral to obtain a larger loan from a micro-credit body.

Savings groups form social capital as well as financial capital

Clearly the main requirement for success in this form of savings is trust between the group members. If someone does not pay in his or her share then the whole thing falls apart. But the main advantage is that it does not rely on outside sources of cash. It also promotes the development of human and social capital, as well as financial capital, because people must be disciplined and they must be strong and cohesive as a group. Most importantly the group members build up a credit record, demonstrating that they are capable of helping themselves and can save, however small an amount. A micro-finance organisation is more likely to look favourably on applicants with this kind of record.

Families can help a disabled person start saving

But again, disabled people start with a disadvantage. If they are not earning anything at all, where will they get the money from to pay in their contribution? It is here that involving the whole nuclear family and perhaps the wider extended family may be important. Another family member may be able to contribute until the disabled person starts earning.

The importance of role models

Additionally, disabled people may be too scattered to form such a group, or not be accepted into a mixed group. This is where role models become very important. Role models of disabled people succeeding in business are present in many communities, and the task of a CBR programme is to find them and make them known, in order to convince both disabled and non-disabled doubters that disabled people are as capable as anybody else, and can be fully contributing members of a mixed group.

Membership of a savings group is also an important mechanism of support for the individual entrepreneur; this is dealt with in detail in Section 10.

SUMMARY

1. Micro-credit is widely used as a development tool but access to mainstream programmes remains difficult for many disabled people.

2. With or without access to micro-credit, savings are an important part of building both financial and social capital, and must be built into any loan programme. A variety of savings methods are possible.

3. Group savings schemes in self-help groups have become the dominant development tool for community development in India, including with disabled people. But in other countries they have not been successful. Trust is a key element in their success.

9. ACCESS TO JOBS IN THE FORMAL ECONOMY

"Create links; build bridges; go out and meet people; be continuously proactive."

Sylvana Lakis, director of LPHU, Lebanon

EXAMPLES FROM JORDAN, LEBANON AND SOUTH AFRICA

Even if pro-disability employment legislation is in place, the reality in many developing countries is that employers in the formal economy do not readily seek to hire disabled people. Programmes aiming at the economic empowerment of disabled people need to be proactive in seeking out possible employers, and not leave it simply to chance. Three examples are given here of organisations which have successfully done this.

The Holy Land Institute for the Deaf in Jordan (HLID) has two types of graduates: those with vocational qualifications, and those capable of going to university and competing as white-collar professionals. With both types the school has adopted a policy of building links with potential employers. For the vocational graduates it is the hotel industry. One case study illustrates the result:

Shaker Hdib is a Palestinian refugee living in Baqa'a refugee camp about 20 minutes' drive north of Amman. Born in 1973, he was deaf from birth. He was one of seven children, three of whom are deaf including him.

To begin with, his parents sought cures and consulted many doctors. At five years old they sent him to HLID, where he remained through to ninth grade, which was as far as the school went then. On finishing ninth grade he joined the vocational training school and learnt carpentry, graduating with a certificate.

In 1998, through the proactive policy adopted by the school targeting the hotel industry, he got a job as maintenance man at the Regency Palace, a five star hotel in Amman. His duties include fixing electrical items, painting, mending and carpentry.

He has good relations with the staff, though communication is difficult. The hotel is very happy with his work, has a high regard for his dependability and good nature and would like to hire more graduates of HLID. They say it is probably the best vocational training school in the country.

His wife is not deaf but they communicate in sign. They have two children who are both hearing.

The Lebanese Physically Handicapped Union (LPHU) has established a wide range of key contacts in so-called 'creative industries' that have enabled disabled people to get jobs as a film archivist, an architectural model maker, and a journalist.

In South Africa, Disabled People of South Africa (DPSA) has worked particularly on the South African Revenue Service (SARS) to ensure that they hire disabled people and this targeted lobbying has paid off. SARS has recently recruited a significant number of disabled persons, several of whom were interviewed for this project. Cynthia Gugu Jelle is a wheelchair user at the Swazi border post.

Born in 1970, she contracted severe polio at 2 and is unable to walk. She attended Ezbeleni special school for physical impairments, a residential school. Her mother worked in Johannesburg as a domestic worker and she only saw her during holidays.

She then attended a government secondary school in Pretoria, which she found exciting and challenging. After graduating she attended Renbeck Access College for disabled persons where she learnt book keeping.

From 1991-8 she stayed at home and had a child.

In 1998 she was employed by Disabled People of South Africa (DPSA) as a provincial administrator. In this role she began to believe in herself as a person, and to develop. Her family began to look up to her because she was earning a wage.

Cynthia says: *"DPSA empowered me as a disabled person. I now know my rights. I can en-courage and empower other people. I developed skills, especially in administration and office work. I am now competitive on the open market."*

In 2002 she studied public relations and administration for six months, sponsored by DPSA.

In June 2004 she got an email from DPSA asking for disabled persons with matric to come forward for jobs with SARS. So she applied and was appointed as a data inputer. SARS provides free accommodation within reach of the border post and transport.

She says: *"I am very happy in this job. I wanted to take the skills I had learnt in DPSA into the world outside disability. I wanted to stretch my wings. SARS needs to learn more about hiring disabled people and is willing to learn. SARS, as a government agency, provides security – job wise and financially. DPSA could not do that.*

'In order to learn one must make mistakes. I am learning to engage with SARS and to help them understand. But I want to work beyond being a team support member. SARS does provide training and I have a very supportive superviser. I need 5000 rand ($820) to repair my electric wheelchair, and SARS is fundraising for this.

'I would like to say to all disabled people: come out! DPSA is there to empower, not protect. Have courage. Don't be negative towards people. People are willing to learn."

In the cases quoted in Jordan, Lebanon and South Africa, targeted lobbying to find a way into the job market for disabled people is effective. This kind of approach requires skills from both the disabled person and the organisation managers.

SUMMARY

1. Placing disabled people in jobs in the formal sector cannot be left to goodwill and legislation. Targeted lobbying and the building of strategic partnerships and alliances with potential employers are required.

2. Primary, secondary and perhaps tertiary education is the key to jobs in the formal sector. Preparation of disabled people for jobs in this sector must therefore start with a focus on education.

10. THE IMPORTANCE OF SUPPORT STRUCTURES

"My strength comes from the group." Sharda, member of disability self-help group, India

GENERATING NETWORKS OF SUPPORT

Support is needed at different levels throughout the life of anybody struggling to survive in a harsh world, and obviously disabled people need it especially. At the most minimal level, support means knowing that you are not alone in your struggles. At more sophisticated levels it means establishing relationships of creative cooperation with a variety of people and groups who work together to solve collective and individual problems. The most successful entrepreneurs will be part of a whole network of community groups of various kinds: savings groups, church groups, a local NGO, perhaps a local council. They are likely to be active promoters of other people's welfare and success as well as their own.

Opha Ndhlovu, a fruit seller in Bulawayo market and a wheelchair user, is an excellent example.

Opha is a wheelchair user aged 35. She was married but her husband deserted her. She has no children of her own, but looks after a niece aged 13. She attended school up to Standard 3, but dropped out because her parents were unable to afford school fees. She now pays school fees for her niece, amounting to some $70 a year.

She was given a loan in 1997 of $30 to start a fruit stall. She makes about $50 a month, selling bananas, apples, oranges and cabbages in the market. She buys from a wholesaler, transporting one crate at a time on her lap in the wheelchair. The price of her bananas was twice as high as her neighbour's. She said she depended on a regular clientele of customers, who always bought from her, so the price was not important.

She has attended a training course in small business management. There she learnt how to manage cash flow, pricing, bookkeeping and customer relations.

She belongs to a range of community groups:

- A women's group
- Seventh Day Adventist Church
- A small savings group using the 'merry-go-round' system
- Resident's association

In all of these groups she is involved in some kind of savings. In the women's group she contributes to a 'burial club'; each member contributes between $0.90 to $1.25 per month. When she dies, her dependent niece will get a lump sum of about $90. This could be used either for funeral costs or for other things.

In her church she belongs to a savings group focused on saving for household items. Each member puts in $0.50 a week, and they take it in turns to 'scoop the pot' in order to buy some necessity for the home.

The larger savings group is a group of 5 friends who each put in $1.80 per week. Every five weeks she gets the $9 which she uses to buy fruit wholesale. (This is essentially a system for helping her cash flow. She buys the fruit wholesale every second or third day, but the extra amount every five weeks enables her to stock more at those intervals.)

In the residents association she contributes to a fund for funerals.

Opha has not noticed any negative attitudes towards her as a disabled person. She has a very outgoing, friendly, positive personality. Her membership of the different groups and circles means that she is both being supported in her life and supporting others. She is a valued member of the community.

Opha says: *"I fear God. I do not use money recklessly. I have an eye for detail. I make friends with my customers. I am active in the community and support others. If I am regarded as successful it is because of these things."*

Opha is an impressive person. She represents the best of survival strategies in poor communities. The most important learning point in her story is not that she sells fruit (in itself a mundane activity), but that she organises her life around a number of networks which support and enrich her life, and which she also enriches with her presence. Her relations with customers are the key to her success in business, and her high reputation in the community means that she has many friends.

SELF-HELP GROUPS

The idea that personal development is closely connected with community development is embodied in the concept of the self-help group (SHG).

The SHG is the dominant mechanism for grassroots development in India, and has been adopted by CBR programmes almost universally in both rural and urban areas.

Some encourage the formation of disability-only SHGs; others encourage mixed non-disabled and disabled membership in SHGs.

The usual aims of these groups are: to give members mutual support for problems shared, to try to solve individual problems, to obtain benefits from the government accorded to them under the law (especially the allocation of 3% of the local budget), and to build group savings.

The way SHGs are used for development in India is impressive. It means that decision-making, practical action, and activism is placed largely in the hands of the target group. The most important lesson for disabled people is that SHGs underline the principle that overcoming isolation and exclusion means pro-actively going out and working with others for the common good and to help other disabled individuals. It is the ultimate blow against sitting at home and waiting for charity.

A further significant advantage of the SHG approach is that it greatly reduces the number of CBR field workers required, and so creates an inherently sustainable programme in a way that is probably unrivalled anywhere else. One CBR worker in a slum area is sufficient if he or she works primarily through SHGs.

There are however two caveats about SHGs that must be expressed in relation to CBR programmes (fully acknowledged by the Indian NGOs themselves). The first is: who owns the groups? The NGO, or are they independent? This is of particular importance when it comes to economic enterprises.

The second is that using SHGs as a CBR strategy to lobby for the provision of rights under the law only works if physical rehabilitation services in particular are actually available. In practice, especially in remote areas, they may not be available, or there may be impossible travel costs and logistical problems for access. In the view of a very experienced occupational therapist heading the CBR programme of the Spastics Society of Karnataka in Bangalore, CBR in India has gone too far in the social model, and neglected the medical aspects of rehabilitation. In his opinion, making SHGs the main medium for CBR means that knowledge about the technicalities of rehabilitation is weak, with the result that important preventive work, early detection, and especially attention to complex impairments like cerebral palsy, are missing or weak.

Despite these drawbacks, the model of SHGs used in India is highly sustainable and comes closer than any other model to the principle of placing responsibility for action in the hands of the target group, and is thus immensely empowering.

In addition, one of the most important tasks in combating poverty is to solve the problem of indebtedness, and it is here that SHGs have most proved their value. Unlike the Grameen Bank model of group guaranteed loans on which community development in Bangladesh is largely based, the Indian SHG model does not rely on outside funds.

There is little doubt that the scale and amount of capital generated through the SHG system, in addition to the powerful sense of group solidarity and mutual support they foster, has made substantial differences to the lives of many poor disabled people in India. These groups have laid the foundations for a powerful movement of disabled people that is genuinely based in the grassroots.

SUMMARY

1. Networks of support are vital to the economic empowerment of disabled people. Disabled people who are most successful, not only in business but in their lives, are those who are members of community groups of various kinds.

2. The self-help group has become the dominant model for community development in India, and is now used by most Indian CBR programmes. This model places responsibility for action in the hands of the target group, and is thus both effective and empowering. Its drawback is that it is weak on physical rehabilitation.

II. CONCLUSIONS: POINTERS FOR ACTION

ENGAGE WITH THE ISSUE

Disabled people usually place economic empowerment as a first priority, with rehabilitation well down the list. But disability programmes tend to be led and staffed by people with a rehabilitation background, who focus on impairment rehabilitation issues. These are important, but employment is, in the eyes of disabled people, more important. So disability programmes need to take the issue of employment support seriously and study it, both theoretically and in their own context. Staff at all levels, from front-line field workers to senior managers, need to have a comprehensive and realistic grasp of the issues surrounding disability, poverty, development and employment.

MAINSTREAM

It will be clear that nearly all the principles about employment support promoted in this paper apply to non-disabled as well as disabled people. The main difference between disabled people and non-disabled is not the impairment but the low expectations in which disabled people are stuck. The main challenge is how to raise these expectations. The key is to mainstream as far as possible, so that disabled people can be part of the same range of expectations as everyone else. This means building links with mainstream development organisations to ensure that disabled people are channelled wherever possible into skills training courses and especially into micro-credit programmes offered for non-disabled people.

RELATE DISABILITY TO OTHER DEVELOPMENT ISSUES

Mainstreaming also means linking disability with other development issues, especially rural development. Disabled groups, because they have strong reasons for mutual self-support, can be pioneers in such innovations as mushroom farming, biogas from cows and high standards of livestock production. Integration is about not focusing on the disability but on the contribution disabled people can make to their own communities. Building links with non-disability organisations such as consumer pressure groups is an important part of the process of creating better conditions for disabled people in employment.

SEEK OUT AND USE ROLE MODELS

Core life skills need to be the focus of all economic empowerment programmes. These skills are directly related to personal empowerment. A change in attitudes must start with disabled people themselves. Disability programmes need to seek out disabled people who show the characteristics of being empowered and use them as role models in training sessions and in other ways.

REFERENCES

Albu, M., 2005. *Improving Business Development Services with Disabled People in Northern Uganda. Evaluation of an action-research project by NUDIPU and APT Enterprise Development.* Available from: http://www.norrag.org/wg/documents/Empowerment%20of%20Disabled.doc

Coleridge, P., 2005. *How do disabled people gain vocational skills and work in community based programmes? Preliminary findings in Africa and the Middle East.* (Unpublished internal report for ILO).

Coleridge, P., in press for 2006. CBR as part of Community Development and Poverty Reduction. In Hartley, S. (ed.) *CBR Africa Regional Conference, Lilongwe, Malawi, August 31 – September 3, 2004.* Norwich: School of Allied Health Professions.

Culshaw, M., 1985. *Vocational Rehabilitation and Integration of the Disabled into the Life of Communities.* ILO (unpublished internal report).

Haan, HC [no date]. *Training for work in the Informal Sector, New evidence from Kenya, Tanzania and Uganda* [online]. ILO. Available from: http://www.ilo.org/ public/english/employment/skills/life/publ/index.htm

ILO, 2002. *Disability and Poverty Reduction Strategies.* Geneva: ILO.

ILO, 2003. *Employment of People with Disabilities: The Impact of Legislation (Asia and the Pacific) Project Consultation Report.* Geneva: ILO

ILO, 2004. *Recommendation* 195. Adopted by the Conference at Its Ninety-Second Session, Geneva, 17 June 2004. Available from: http://www.logos-net. net/ilo/195_base/en/rec/rec_b.htm

Klugman, J. (ed), 2001. *Sourcebook to the PRSP Process.* Washington: World Bank.

Metts, R., Metts N., Oleson T., Dotson-Etcheverria T., 1993. *Report on the Disabled Persons Loan Scheme of Project KEN/86/037.* New York: Cornell University.

Ram, R. & Harris-White, B., 1995. Public sector employment policy and the constitutional and legal vulnerability of physically disabled people in India. *Actionaid Disability News, 6 (2).*

Satish, G., 2001. Questioning the 'Rights-Based' Approach. *Nav Bharat Jagriti Kendra News, April-June 2001 issue.*

World Bank, 2004. *Global Partnership for Disability and Development, Declaration of Purpose.* Available from: http://siteresources.worldbank.org/DISABILITY/ Resources/News---Events/GPDD/DeclarationFinal2005.doc

CHAPTER 5

CONFLICT RECOVERY

DR MARIA KETT

I. INTRODUCTION

The impact of disasters and conflicts on disabled people's lives affects how programmes in the other areas of Leonard Cheshire International's work – economic empowerment, inclusive education, and inclusive community service – are implemented. Despite the increasing frequency and complexity of modern conflicts and disasters, there is still very little research on the links between disability, disasters and conflicts. Nor is there very much evidence of the inclusion of disabled people at any stage of recovery, from emergency interventions through to longer term development.

Using specific examples, this paper will focus on the longer-term impacts rather than the immediate post-disaster or post-conflict phases, in line with the author's experiences. It will also serve to illustrate how the exclusion of disabled people in the immediate phase has long term repercussions. Finally, the paper will look at some of the ways in which the barriers to inclusion and participation can be overcome.

The paper contextualises disability, conflict and disasters within current debates. Many of the issues discussed within it, for example the links between poverty, inequality and conflict, cut across societies and cultures, countries and continents. But the paper highlights the exclusionary mechanisms these have resulted in for disabled people, some of the ways they have been overcome, and what more needs to be done for genuinely participatory, inclusive development in conflict and disaster-affected areas around the world.

The paper is based on research undertaken by the Leonard Cheshire Centre of Conflict Recovery (LCC), a department of LCI based at University College London.

2. DISABILITY, CONFLICT AND DISASTERS

Modern conflicts are increasingly complex, and asymmetric, fought not between conventional armies, but between groups where the 'enemy' may be invisible and not abiding by any conventional rules of war. This means that civilians are now the most common casualties of conflict (around 9:1). The statistics make for terrible reading in Rwanda, over 500,000 people have missing limbs and over 300,000 people have impairments from wounds sustained during the genocide (Jones 2006). Advances in medical technology have led to people surviving injuries they previously would have·not. However survival may mean lifelong impairment and subsequent disability. For example, serious injuries may require long-term medical intervention. This can be costly and can have severe repercussions on affected individuals and their families. These can include difficulties with housing, food, education and clothing. All of these can further result in poverty and social exclusion.

Conflict, disasters and disability are not only linked directly through injuries or accidents, but also more indirect effects such as inadequate healthcare, poverty, and malnutrition (Murray et al. 2002). Conflict-related injuries put additional strain on healthcare resources in already severely overstretched countries. Consequently, disabled people are often a low priority in service provision, furthering isolation and marginalisation. In the aftermath of a conflict or disaster, people with pre-existing impairments may find their often already precarious situation exacerbated by the loss of family members or carers, moving to temporary housing or shelter, loss of mobility and other aids, and difficulty in accessing information, food, water or sanitation sources and lack of other infrastructure (Edmonds 2005). Yet the WHO estimates that five to seven per cent of people in camps or temporary shelters following a disaster have a disability.[15]

Inevitably, anyone affected by disasters or conflict may also be vulnerable to psychological sequelae, including emotional distress and mental health problems (MSF 1997). One third to one half of all people affected by disasters show some symptoms of post-traumatic stress and related distress (WHO 2001). People with mental health problems often experience the worst forms of discrimination, abuse of human rights and exclusion at all levels of society. Mental health services are particularly under-resourced, staffed, and funded and though there is an increasing focus on the provision of psychosocial programmes by both local and international agencies (van Ommeren et al. 2005), there remains a discrepancy between a focus on (psychosocial) trauma and wider mental health issues.

According to the WHO, conflict-related injuries and disabilities account for some 4.8 million Disability Adjusted Life Years worldwide.[16] UNICEF estimates that for every child killed, three are permanently impaired.[17] Of those that survive injuries, access to medical care, prosthetics and rehabilitation is extremely limited, despite the growing demand. It is estimated that only 5 to 15 per cent of the population can access any kind of assistive technology in many developing countries (WHO 2006).

In emergency situations disabled people sustain disproportionately higher rates of morbidity and mortality, yet are often the most excluded and least able to access emergency aid. Many disabled people are left behind when a disaster strikes a community. For those lucky enough to actually make it to relief centres or camps, there may be difficulties with emergency registration systems or relief efforts. Other disabling factors include the loss of support structures (including family members), loss of mobility and accessibility aids, and change in terrain or location, including refugee camps. Both disabled and non-disabled people are susceptible to (further) impairments through lack of medical care, loss of infrastructure, lack of rehabilitation facilities, poverty, poor nutrition, and lack of maternal and child healthcare (e.g. vaccination campaigns). Disabled people, especially women and children, are particularly vulnerable to violence, exploitation and sexual abuse (Boyce 2000; Harris and Enfield 2003). Women often bear the brunt of conflict, losing members of their families and becoming head of household, having to care for children as well as the infirm, yet there is often little precious support for women or children in these situations. Overall, the diversity of disabled people is very often ignored – in particular the gendered and generational aspects of injury and disability (World Bank 2005a). Programmes often ignore local requirements, for example the differing needs of urban and rural communities.

Once infrastructures such as healthcare systems are destroyed, they can take years to regenerate. The effects are demonstrable across indicators such as maternal and child mortality rates, nutrition, and infectious diseases (especially HIV/AIDS).

---

[15] Resource Paper/Lobbying Tool-Kit on 'DEVELOPMENT ISSUES - particularly International Cooperation –in the context of the Draft Comprehensive and Integral International Convention on the Rights and Dignity of Persons with Disabilities' IDDC UN Convention Task Group June 9, 2006

[16] The sum of years of potential life lost due to premature mortality and the years of productive life lost due to disability (http://www.who.int/disabilities/en/)

[17] Resource Paper/Lobbying Tool-Kit on 'DEVELOPMENT ISSUES - particularly International Cooperation –in the context of the Draft Comprehensive and Integral International Convention on the Rights and Dignity of Persons with Disabilities' IDDC UN Convention Task Group June 9, 2006

There are chronic shortages of access to food, water, sewerage and utilities; fear and threats to physical security. Communicable diseases and psychological distress are commonplace, as are injuries from antipersonnel mines, firearms and other violent acts (Banatvala and Zwi 2000; Murray et al. 2002, Kett and Mannion 2004). Both disasters and conflicts result in movement of people. Women, children and the elderly make up the majority of refugee and displaced populations as male family members are left behind to fight, or are killed in the process. Internally displaced people (IDPs) forced to migrate as a result of conflict have not crossed international borders, and consequently are not protected by international laws, unlike refugees. Refugees and IDPs face challenges of hunger, inadequate shelter, poverty, psychological stress, epidemics, and are subsequently more at risk from 'natural' disasters such as famine. Of the 25 million people displaced across 52 countries most are in Africa, with some 13 million people displaced largely as a result of conflicts across the continent.[18] Many end up living in temporary camps and shelters for years. There has been very little research into the specific needs of disabled people in situations of migration and displacement.

It is not just conflict situations that have become increasingly complex. Due to the inevitable political influences many seemingly 'natural' disasters have become increasingly complex humanitarian emergencies (CHEs) – complex in both nature and solution. There is currently much debate about the politics of aid and humanitarian relief and intervention, and there have been a number of examples of notable failures in international humanitarian interventions, in particular Rwanda and Bosnia.

It may also be the case, as happened in Sri Lanka and Indonesia when the Indian Ocean Tsunami hit on December 2004, that the impact of the disaster overlaps with the effects of already-existing conflict, with differing outcomes and responses. This is because areas affected by conflict are invariably poorer, with weaker social structures to begin with. Communities living in poverty also tend to suffer more from natural disasters: they lack early warning systems, have weaker infrastructure and have fewer resources for recovery. In the aftermath of the Indian Ocean Tsunami in December 2004, it is estimated that across the Asia Pacific region, the number of disabled people increased by 20 per cent (World Bank 2005b).

Despite the evidence that disabled people are one of the most affected groups in disasters, and that emergency responses are inadequate to reach out to disabled people (Parr 1987), disabled people have largely been excluded from post-conflict and post-disaster relief and development programmes – from the mitigation and planning stages right through to longer term development programmes (Kett et al. 2005). Though one of the most decisive factors in this exclusion is poverty, it is not just poor countries that exclude disabled people from emergency relief and rehabilitation programmes. Following Hurricane Katrina in the USA, there were numerous reports of disabled people being ignored and excluded in federal relief and rescue programmes (NOD).

Poverty is a major driving force for war and conflict, for example over scarce or valuable resources, or inequalities. The increased complexity of such conflicts means there is often no clear beginning, middle and end. Modern 'low intensity' conflicts may grind on for years, and result in a lack of human security; chronic poverty from the decimated infrastructure and industry and subsequent unemployment; loss of land and housing; limited access to schools, healthcare facilities and other welfare structures. As a result of these circumstances, many people become dependent on external aid, which combined with ongoing resource scarcity and inequalities, may in turn foster further conflicts.

Strategies for survival and recovery vary according to a number of factors, and include security, ability, financial wherewithal, dependants, family commitments, opportunities, sense of attachment and belonging, justice, peace, security and reconciliation. Despite the prevalence of conflict-related impairments, it is not physical impairments that hamper reconstruction and development, but how people are excluded from these processes, as examples from Sierra Leone and Sri Lanka in this paper will demonstrate. By reversing the processes of exclusion, disabled people can become involved in efforts to reconstruct countries affected by conflict, not only contributing to the reconstruction, but also the rehabilitation of the country.

Whilst disabled people are rarely prioritised in relief or development interventions, the collapse of basic infrastructures, family displacement, and lack of awareness, know-ledge and skills in mainstream emergency/relief agencies undermines the

---

[18] The Global IDP Project (http://www.idpproject.org/)

potential for disabled persons to participate and access their basic rights. This is further exacerbated by a tendency to treat disabled people as passive victims. Even if there are national and international legislations nominally in place, disabled people are often excluded in practice, for example, due to gaps in policy implementation between urban and rural areas, or between areas affected by conflict and those not (Kett et al. 2005).

3. THE RIGHTS-BASED APPROACH TO HUMANITARIAN AID AND DEVELOPMENT

Most international non-government organisations (INGOs) and UN agencies promote a rights-based approach to aid and development. This has particular saliency for 'vulnerable groups'. Like gender, disability is a cross-cutting issue; yet when disabled people are included (as a vulnerable group), they are often seen as requiring specialist intervention, rather than lacking rights. Addressing fundamental issues of rights, inclusion and equality are effective ways of tackling vulnerability in itself. Disabled people require many of the same support structures, aid and interventions as may other sections of the population, such as the elderly, children, pregnant women and people living with HIV/AIDS. For example, the basic needs in immediate post-emergency phases are the same for all – water, shelter, food, sanitation etc. It is how they are provided that makes the difference. Nevertheless, few programmes take into account the specific needs of disabled people in such situations, despite some attempts to ameliorate this, for example the Sphere Guidelines – though not until the revised 4th edition (The Sphere Project 2004). However, these are only meant as guidelines, focusing primarily on immediate measures and responses. In addition, a number of INGOs working in the area of disability and development have begun collating their experience, and drafted specific guidelines: these include guidelines on accessible reconstruction and water and sanitation a list of which can be found on the World Bank website.[19] There is very little in the way of guidelines for inclusive medium to longer term recovery and rehabilitation projects, and few examples of disability programmes being included in poverty reduction strategies (Inclusion International 2005, Edmonds 2005). This is a particularly important area, especially as the timeline between emergencies and longer term rehabilitation is blurred, thus increasing the risk of exclusion.

Many international NGOs and local NGOs now incorporate the language of the social model of disability into their programmes, advocating an inclusive,

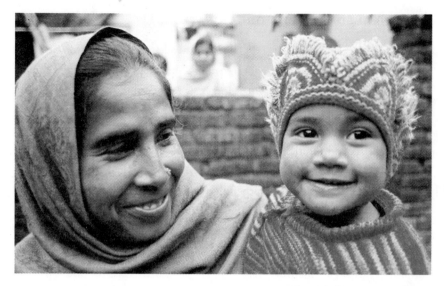

participatory model in both emergency relief and longer term development. However, this is often counteracted by practices on the ground (Kett et al. 2005). Though a number of policies and guidelines exist, it remains a challenge to operationalise them in ways that are genuinely participatory and inclusive, whereby disabled people are included – not just consulted – at all phases of the planning and intervention cycle, from mitigation and emergency relief, to longer-term reconstruction and rehabilitation plans. Inclusive policies and practices can also be more cost-effective if undertaken from the beginning rather than implemented at a later stage, for example, reconstructing accessible buildings.

There are a number of measures which can be taken to promote meaningful participation and inclusion of disabled people in post-disaster and post-conflict relief and development programmes. First and foremost of these is the inclusion and participation of disabled people themselves at all stages of planning and programming. Disabled people are aware of their own specific needs, particularly the cultural and social context, and can work with programmes to ensure adequate representation and training is undertaken. One way that has been particularly beneficial is working through disabled people's organisations (DPOs).

---

[19] http://www.dgroups.org/groups/worldbank/Disaster-Disability/index.cfm

3.1 DISABLED PEOPLE'S ORGANISATIONS

Disabled people's organisations (DPOs) can act as advocates or mediators and are a crucial component to ensure the inclusion of disabled people in disaster and conflict recovery planning and programming. The crisis in the acute stages of conflict, or the aftermath of a disaster, can act as a catalyst for the formation of self-help groups and DPOs, as examples below will demonstrate. However, the development of these potential opportunities, as well as the support for more specific campaigns for accessibility and inclusion can be challenging. Among the many problems small-scale NGOs and DPOs face are recognition and access to donor funding – unless they work in partnership with larger (international) organisations already known to the donors these may be difficult. However, there is a danger that this can perpetuate the view that disabled people are unable to speak for themselves, by both the organisation, and the donors. It is also vital for DPOs to make links with other civil society organisations and movements to ensure that the voices of disabled people are heard by governments, ministries and other forums, and to engage with wider global movements such as that to alleviate poverty.

It is important to remember that not every disabled person belongs to a disabled people's organisation, nor has access to information about what resources are available for them, especially in the chaotic aftermath of a large disaster. This is particularly the case for disabled children and young adults, who may have differing needs to their families. Disabled people are not one homogeneous group, and there is of course diversity. Differences may arise from impairment, gender, age, geographical location, whether or not the person became disabled as a result of conflict, or was already disabled, as well as whether problems were exacerbated by the disaster or conflict i.e. through lack of healthcare, malnutrition, or loss of support structures. In many conflict-affected countries, war-related disability raises politically and economically difficult issues such as compensation. Differences and diversity also highlight the issue of prioritising and defining disability, especially those often excluded, for example children with intellectual impairment, or people with mental health problems. The diversity of disabled people and their differing needs must be taken into consideration to ensure that disabled people are genuinely at the core of programmes and policies in this field.

3.2 INCLUSION AT DONOR LEVEL

Disability in situations of disaster and emergency is also prioritised by a number of international organisations, particularly those working in the field of disability and development.[20] Though it is increasingly coming to the attention of mainstream organisations, it is often as a 'vulnerable' group. Moreover, it remains a continuing challenge to actually operationalise already-existing policies and practices in the field. This is due to a number of barriers, including lack of awareness and training, funding and representation. There is also limited acknowledgement of the role of DPOs in the field, and as noted above, many international donors and organisations do not work with or through local DPOs. This may unintentionally perpetuate exclusion, especially at national level, if DPOs are not prioritised.

Perhaps as a result of the number of disasters that occurred throughout 2005, including the Indian Ocean Tsunami, Hurricane Katrina in the USA and the Pakistan earthquake, there are currently a number of initiatives and policies regarding inclusive policies in situations of conflict and emergencies being instigated. It is these that most funding lines for projects and programmes are based on, and for the sake of brevity, listed below are just a selection of some of the inclusive policies, guidelines and initiatives agencies have drafted.

In 1996, UNHCR published a manual aiming to promote the inclusion of disabled refugees at the community level (UNHCR 1996). The three parts of the manual help to make a first assessment, to plan preventive measures and to establish rehabilitation. UNHCR considers disabled people a 'priority group', especially in situations of displacement and resettlement; that is, they will be amongst the first to be included in mainstream programmes. In such circumstances, UNHCR does relief work and refers onto appropriate local and international agencies.

UNICEF too has guidelines for inclusion of disabled children in complex humanitarian emergencies, specifically through child protection mandates (which vary according to country). Disability is mainstreamed as a cross cutting issue within other focus groups, for example, children and women. Other UN agencies, including UNESCAP and UNDP have specific policies regarding disability. The proposed UN Convention on the Rights and Dignity of Persons with Disabilities may also assist

---

[20] See for example the International Disability and Development Consortium. http://www.iddc.org.uk/

with this process – though it is important to remember that many member-countries do not have any specific disability legislation. There are plans for a specific article (Article 11) on 'People in Situations of Risk'. This non-contentious wording allows for some scope to lobby for the rights of disabled people in emergency situations, particularly protection; reintegration; accessibility; and disaster preparedness.[21]

The WHO has shifted focus from the purely medical aspects of disability – though in-country, they are mandated to work through national health services and governments wherever possible. The WHO has a number of departments focusing specifically on disability issues: the Disability and Rehabilitation Team (DAR); the Department of Injuries and Violence Prevention (VIP), which looks at injury-related disability and rehabilitation; and the Department for Non-communicable Diseases and Mental Health. These incorporate work on disasters and conflicts within the teams. For example, following the tsunami the WHO set up a site devoted to 'Injuries and disability: priorities and management for populations affected by the earthquake and tsunami in Asia', which describes the most appropriate medical interventions for people injured as a result of the tsunami.[22] The WHO is currently in the process of redrafting the Guidelines for Community Based Rehabilitation (CBR), which will include specific guidelines for CBR in crisis situations.

Some other international legislation that can be used to support right-based approaches in post-conflict and post-disaster planning and programming includes the UN Convention on the Rights of the Child, UN Convention on the Elimination of All Forms of Discrimination against Women, UN Standard Rules on the Equalization of Opportunities for Persons with Disabilities, as well as a number of other International Statutes and Humanitarian Laws.

Some bilateral donor organisations have specific departments on disability – for example the Disability and Development team at the World Bank. Early in 2006, the World Bank funded an e-forum on Disability and Natural Disasters, which drew participants from around the world into discussions highlighting examples of good and bad practice, linking groups and creating all kinds of new networks and collaborations, as well as really getting the issue onto the agenda of the international donor agencies.[23]

USAID has what at first sight appears to be a fairly comprehensive policy for inclusion;[24] however, in the field it is often tied to so many conditions that much of it becomes difficult to implement. For example, USAID does not directly fund any programmes, but provides small grants – usually to civil society organisations – by way of goods or services, for example to support livelihood programmes, infrastructure repairs or access to information. This funding is contingent on location and (political) affiliation. In emergency relief programmes, the USAID policy of paying beneficiaries cash for work effectively discriminates against those who for any number of reasons are unable to work (it should be noted that this method of involving beneficiaries on programmes is not unique to USAID).

In the UK, DFID focuses on mainstreaming disability as part of its commitment to a rights based approach and the eradication of social exclusion. They support meaningful consultation and inclusion of disabled people at all stages of planning and implementation of activities. DFID advocates the twin track approach – addressing disability within all strategic areas of work, whilst at the same time supporting specific initiatives to empower disabled people.[25]

So there is some (theoretical) commitment to addressing the specific needs of disabled people by international donor organisations. As noted above, without taking these into consideration disabled people will continue to be excluded from mainstream development programmes. Of course, how disability is addressed within countries depends very much on local context and legislations. Overcoming barriers to exclusion also depends on a number of other factors: disabled people being treated as equals, with the same rights and needs as everyone else in society; changing attitudes; positive role models; funding for disabled people and their organisations, and meaningful consultations and dialogue. Much of this work is undertaken at community level. There has been a great deal of discussion around the importance of community based rehabilitation (CBR) programmes in countries affected by conflict and disasters as relatively cost-effective, local methods to facilitate inclusion.

[21] Resource Paper/Lobbying Tool-Kit on 'DEVELOPMENT ISSUES - particularly International Cooperation –in the context of the Draft Comprehensive and Integral International Convention on the Rights and Dignity of Persons with Disabilities' IDDC UN Convention Task Group June 9, 2006

[22] http://www.who.int/violence_injury_prevention/other_injury/tsunami/en/index.html

[23] http://www.dgroups.org/groups/worldbank/Disaster-Disability/index.cfm

[24] http://www.usaid.gov/about/disability/

[25] http://www.dfid.gov.uk/news/files/devawareness/disability-day.asp

4. CONFLICT, DISASTERS AND COMMUNITY-BASED SERVICES

It has been estimated that 80 per cent of the information, skills, and resources that disabled people need to enable them to fully participate and access their rights can be met within their local communities. However, to be fully effective, this entails governments taking the responsibility to ensure that disabled people are in a position to do so, and that accessible, affordable, relevant services are available in these communities (IDDC 2000). Whilst on the one hand, abdicating responsibility to the community allows disabled people within these communities a degree of autonomy, it is important to ascertain what community-level priorities are – they may not be consistent with broader development goals of equity, efficiency and sustainability, nor with disabled people themselves.

Community based approaches are increasingly important in post-conflict and post-disaster settings as a tool to deliver early rehabilitation and provision of basic goods and services,[26] though a recent discussion paper highlighted the potential pitfalls of implementing them in difficult political environments (Slaymaker et al. 2005). In such areas, states may be weak or non-existent, and lack the resources necessary to engage in countrywide programmes. This has particularly been the case for community-based rehabilitation (CBR) programmes for disabled people.

Responsibility for most CBR projects has been in the hands of those implementing the programmes. This has meant that, until very recently, the involvement of disabled people has been tokenistic, with participation being largely rhetorical and based on donor requirements, perpetuating professional dominance and hierarchal power relations (Finkenflügel 2006). This has had a bearing on how CBR projects have been implemented. While there have been many successful pilot projects, there is a limited evidence-base of examples being scaled up to national service provision level, and a subsequent ongoing lack of resources for training and personnel in many countries affected by disasters or conflict.

Wherever possible, CBR interventions have been shifted from an institution, for example a hospital, to the homes and communities of the disabled person. This facilitates inclusive, community-based interventions that can be carried out by people with minimal training, who typically can be drawn from the disabled person's family or community. It also moves away from a medical approach, which sees the person as a 'problem' to be 'cured', not the negative social attitudes toward the disabled person which are debilitating. The social model does not reject medical intervention or assistive devices per se – indeed, these can be liberating for the disabled person – but does reject the medicalisation of disability. An effective CBR programme also challenges the charity model, in which the disabled person is seen as a 'deserving victim'. Participatory, community-based care is thus empowering and rights-based. Such an approach may also reduce costs; however this does depend on what human and capital resources are available locally, as well as how effective the implementing structures are.

At their best, CBR programmes can be empowering, creating advocates and focal points within communities and raising social responsibility. They can provide support, networks and resources to disabled people and their organisations. CBR increases inclusion and community empowerment and raises awareness and social responsibility. Importantly, CBR programmes can provide links with other activities, for example through the support and creation of DPOs.

However, many CBR programmes are written with an unproblematised concept of 'community'. Not everyone has a sense of belonging to a 'community', or put another way, people may have very different notions of what constitutes a community. Particularly in communities affected by conflict, the very fabric and structure of the 'community' may be broken, damaged or destroyed. Moreover, there has been a strong emphasis on family involvement – with the assumption of homogeneity and harmony. Children have very often been excluded from CBR programmes. In many cases, families, especially women, are too poor and over-burdened to play an active role in programmes (Giacaman 2001). Conversely, in many countries, the concept of community is often regarded more highly than the individual – people are inter-dependent, rather than independent.[27]

There is as yet still little evidence to measure the universality of application of the CBR strategy, or indeed its effectiveness in this field. There has been no evidence that CBR is any more cost-effective than any other method of delivering services, especially in conflict- or disaster-affected areas.

---

[26] 'Potentials and limits of community-based service delivery in post-conflict situations' *id21* 17 February 2006. URL: http://www.id21.org/zinter/id21zinter.exe?a=i&w=s10cts1g1

[27] Similarly, Peter Coleridge notes how in a CBR group in Afghanistan, the word 'empowerment' had little resonance, as it implied a hierarchical value. The group preferred the term 'enablement' – but: ".. even this is a concept not easily understood in a situation where people may not aspire to individual development at all, imbued with cultural values that are dominated by the need for collective family survival and kin-group solidarity" (Coleridge 1998).

CBR is not an alternative model or approach in conflict or disaster-recovery work; rather it is one approach that can be used in response to the community's needs. There must be appropriate resources and tools available, provided by the government or other organisations. This raises the issues of responsibility, and whether CBR programmes allow national governments to abdicate responsibility for disabled people. Another criticism of CBR programmes is that they are too specialist, therefore they are not included or considered in mainstream programmes – conversely, some reports have shown that people in CBR programmes may not always get the specialist referrals they need if there are no links with other services (SHIA/WHO 2002). Overall, there needs to be more focus at all levels of society – from central policy makers, disabled people and civil society organisations as well as the wider community – on what their recovery needs are. An example of such an approach is that taken by LCI in its community-based project in Kabala, northern Sierra Leone.

5. COMMUNITY-BASED APPROACHES – CASE STUDY: SIERRA LEONE

LCI have had a presence in Sierra Leone for many years, but since 2001, the West Africa Regional Office (WARO) has been based in Freetown. Attending the monthly co-ordination meeting of NGOs working to rebuild the country after 11 years civil war, the Regional Programme Manager noticed that there was very little information regarding the situation of disabled people, particularly children in the north of the country. Most of the INGOs were concentrating their expertise on the 'war wounded and amputees', a highly visible group of men, women and children who had survived brutal injuries and deliberate maiming during the course of the war. The INGOs were offering rehabilitation services, prosthetics, and psychosocial programmes as well as building resettlement camps for them across the country. However, the majority of non-war disabled were effectively, if unintentionally, excluded from these programmes.

To redress this lack of attention, particularly to children, the WARO initiated a community-based project in conjunction with a number of local DPOs which would enable disabled children to access mainstream primary and secondary level education. The project was implemented in conjunction with moves to create sustainable livelihoods through economic empowerment for young disabled adults too old for formal education programmes, and micro-credit loans for disabled

In conflict-affected countries, war-related disability can raise politically and economically difficult issues such as compensation. The recommendations of the SLTRC are as yet unimplemented by the government, and will potentially be very costly to them. A number of the war amputees the author has met in Sierra Leone have expressed their anger that their perpetrators had probably gone through disarmament, demobilisation and rehabilitation (DDR) programmes, yet they have been left with nothing. But only those directly affected by conflict, such as landmine survivors or amputees, will be eligible if they ever receive the money. For most disabled people, social welfare and support remains limited, and as noted above, large numbers of disabled adults and children resort to living off the streets.

The situation for those not impaired as a result of the conflict is quite dire. There is no legislation regarding disability in Sierra Leone, and apart from the potential compensation for the war wounded, very little in the way of welfare. Yet even for those who were not impaired as a direct result of the conflict, many of the problems they face now are related to the effects of the conflict. These include lack of healthcare (including disruption of mass vaccination campaigns), malnutrition and lack of maternal and child healthcare. Therefore those who were already impaired before the conflict may have become even more disabled as a consequence: families were separated, support structures destroyed, personal items lost, and poverty and fleeing fighting often forced mothers to abandon the children or leave them in places where it was perceived they would be better off, such as residential services. Many of these disabled people have been forgotten or excluded from rehabilitation and reconstruction projects, education and access to employment. This can result in "generations of learned helplessness among disabled refugees ..." (Boyce 2000: 90). Women and children, youth, adults and children with learning disabilities and those with mental health problems, as well as those subjected to institutionalisation are especially excluded (IDDC 2004).

Disabled people in Sierra Leone face numerous barriers to full inclusion in society. The biggest of these is chronic poverty: as a result, disabled people face discrimination in all aspects of society, and as yet there is no national legislation to ameliorate this (though this is currently under review).[31] Disabled children are among those most marginalised and excluded within communities. This may be for any number

---

[31] The Government of Sierra Leone (GoSL) Ministry of Social Welfare, Gender and Children's Affairs is in the process of collaborating with the Law Reform Commission to produce a Law on Disability. However, there is limited funding for a national policy. http://www.statehouse-sl.org/speeches/law-ref-apr8.html

people and parents of disabled children. Before moving on to outline the elem[...]
of the programme, it is necessary to give some background to its development, [...]
to the current context within Sierra Leone.

Despite relative stability and signs of economic recovery in the five years since [...]
signing of the peace agreement in 2001, Sierra Leone was left with familiar legac[...]
of war, and faces a number of ongoing problems primarily related to enden[...]
poverty. These include dilapidated infrastructure, gender inequalities (especially[...]
access to education),[28] poor human resource development, and high unemployme[...]
(especially amongst youth in urban areas). The war and its aftermath have also result[...]
in increasing urbanisation and a concurrent rise of the number of homeless peop[...]
and street children. In Sierra Leone inequality was one of the main contributin[...]
factors to the conflict.[29] The NGO Human Rights Watch have identified the lac[...]
of job opportunities as a major impediment to breaking the cycle of war in West[...]
Africa, which results in "regional warriors" who go from one conflict to another for[...]
money or loot.[30]

As noted above, many people were left deliberately maimed during the course of
the conflict, and following the cessation of hostilities, a large number of INGOs in
Sierra Leone focused specifically on these 'war wounded and amputees'. Now most
of these organisations have left, and although people remain in the resettlement
camps, many report that they feel they have been abandoned with little social
support, unusable prosthesis, few skills and no money. Conversely, by remaining
in the camps their visibility is maintained, as is their voice – particularly important
in lobbying for the compensation recommended by the Sierra Leone Truth and
Reconciliation Commission (SLTRC). So, in most cases they have become a community despite their differences. As international aid and attention shifts, some of
these camp-based organisations are forming their own community organisation[...]
and DPOs. Despite this, many amputees and their children resort to street beggin[...]
as a means of survival. Even if their cases are referred to the Ministry of Soci[...]
Welfare, there is little recourse for them and it becomes increasingly difficult [...]
break this cycle.

---

[28] http://www.unicef.org/infobycountry/sierraleone.html

[29] http://www.irinnews.org/report.asp?ReportID=50827&SelectRegion=West_Africa&SelectCountry=
SIERRA_LEONE

[30] http://www.irinnews.org/report.asp?ReportID=52035&SelectRegion=West_Africa&SelectCountry=GUINEA

of reasons – including fear, stigma, and lack of parental expectations. Disabled children are far more likely than non-disabled children not to attend school, or to have their schooling disrupted or shortened. Some groups in particular are even more marginalised – particularly pre-school-age disabled children, adolescents, and those with learning disabilities and mental health problems. There is anecdotal evidence that, as in many countries, adolescents with learning disabilities may be disproportionably represented in the criminal justice system, and given the lack of juvenile detention centres and courts in Sierra Leone, may not receive fair or adequate trials or treatment. Disabled children and young adults are at risk of violence and abuse – young disabled women are often subjected to rape, or coerced into sex, resulting in high numbers of single parent families and further marginalisation of the women. This has wider implications too, particularly HIV/AIDS.

The most successful projects are those that attempt to break this cycle and remove the barriers that stop disabled people being fully included in society. Overall, there is a wide lack of awareness or knowledge regarding the social model of disability: disabled people (or their impairment) are often seen as being the 'problem', and not the society's attitude toward them. However, mainly as a consequence of poverty, many impairments are not seen so readily as 'curable' (from a medical model perspective), and so it is often the case that innovative solutions are found – often by disabled people themselves – to enable them to participate in society.

As a direct consequence of the conflict, a number of DPOs formed, initially to provide emergency relief and support to disabled people during the war, but have continued to grow in strength in the aftermath. Despite this, many feel excluded from the wider development process. They now mostly advocate and campaign on disability issues, though some also offer skills training, loans and other support. The Sierra Leone Union of Disability Issues (SLUDI) is an umbrella organisation of DPOs and is actively involved in promulgating for reform and creation of national disability legislation that would give disabled people more rights within society. However, disabled children are often ignored by local DPOs – unless the DPO is formed out of a parent group.

An example of one such DPO is the Freetown based Handicap Action Movement (HAM), formed by disabled people who had fled to the capital during the conflict. After intermittent support from NGOs over the years, they are now largely self-sustaining, and undertake training of other disabled people in tool making and carpentry. They recently won a large government contract to make agricultural implements such as machetes. Nevertheless, such programmes should not be assumed to be an acceptable alternative to changing social expectations and attitudes toward disability.

5.1 KABALA COMMUNITY BASED PROGRAMME

LCI advocates a twin track approach to both promote inclusion in mainstream projects, as well as focus on the specific needs of disabled children, such as access. In this way, projects do not focus solely on 'vulnerable' groups, which may inadvertently increase inequalities, but on the whole of the society. The Kabala community-based inclusive education and economic empowerment project in the north of Sierra Leone exemplifies such an approach. Kabala was chosen as it is one of the poorest regions in Sierra Leone, and suffered heavily during the civil conflict. Much of its infrastructure was destroyed. However, families have returned to the area and it is slowly returning to life. To ensure community ownership of the project, a village management committee (VMC) was set up, which includes disabled children and adults participating in the programme. The VMC also links directly with the two regional Paramount Chiefs, the District Council, Ministry of Social Welfare, as well as other NGOs in the area.

It is well acknowledged that enrolling children in education or training programmes promotes a sense of normalcy and inclusion, particularly in conflict-affected situations. In the immediate aftermath of the war, a number of agencies (led by UNICEF) commenced accelerated education programmes that enabled older children (8-18 years) who had missed out on years of primary school education to complete primary school in three years instead of six.[32] However, these programmes were initiated as an emergency measure, and not as part of longer term development strategies, so are in the process of being phased out in order to prevent over-dependency by the state education sector. UNICEF is currently in the process of assessing the effectiveness of these programmes, but it seems that a number of children, particularly older children and girls, have not had the opportunity to undergo these programmes and may have also missed out on other education initiatives. Conversely, many of the Adult Learning Initiatives have focused primarily on women. Arbitrary age limits can mean that a number of people, particularly young adolescents, are excluded from programmes aimed at children, but are not eligible to join adult programmes.

It was imperative that any reintegration programmes were undertaken in conjunction with poverty reduction strategies and community building activities. Direct assistance, in the form of donation of education materials and furniture, as well as enabling physical access through aids such as ramps, was necessary to create the conditions in which all the children in the schools benefit. Many schools were damaged or destroyed during the war and needed repairs, so this was an opportunity to reconstruct the schools in an inclusive way at little extra cost. The local community was involved in providing some of the building material as well as the labour. Teachers were given in-service training relative to the care, inclusion and specific teaching methods for disabled children. The programme includes a 'Training of Trainers' component, so that these teachers can subsequently train colleagues in other schools. The inclusion of a number of children was enhanced through the provision of mobility aids in conjunction with the NGO Mercy Ships/ New Steps, who also provided prosthetics and orthopaedic services for those children who needed them.

It was challenging to provide skills training to the large number of young adults above school age within the community who, after years of disrupted schooling, had high rates of illiteracy. After community consultation, young disabled adults asked for training in basic skills such as blacksmithing, tailoring, hairdressing, and weaving (see Box 1). At the end of the apprenticeship, trainees are provided with starter kits to establish their own small enterprises for independent living. The community project also established a revolving loan scheme which has grown incrementally over the course of the programme, and many women have been enabled to support the education of their children.

---

[32] Such as the Complementary Rapid Education Programmes (CREPs)

BOX I: MOHAMMED'S STORY

Mohammed is 19 years old. He was born in the east of the country not long before the war started. Due to the disruption in public health services, he was not immunised and contracted polio. After his mother was killed, the rest of his family managed to escape to Kabala to stay with his elder sister and her family,

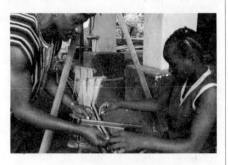

Photo: Jenny Matthews / Leonard Cheshire

until they too decided to flee due to encroaching fighting. They left him behind fearing his restricted mobility would hold them back. He stayed on in Kabala, hiding in the bush whenever the rebel soldiers came through the area. Eventually he moved into another house in the village with a group of friends. He had no formal education, apart from a three month rapid learning programme with an INGO in 2004, and had never had a job. When he met the LCI representative, they discussed his options for skills training. Mohammed expressed a wish to learn the traditional skill of weaving, something that very few other people in Kabala could do at that time. He was sent to Freetown to undergo training, and was elected to be part of the village management committee for the LCI project by the participants at the sensitisation workshop. He returned to Kabala after the three months training and set up his own small enterprise.

The LCI project has bought many benefits to the community in Kabala. In terms of post-conflict recovery, many participating schools have been rebuilt, and are fully accessible and inclusive (see picture 3, page 175). There are a variety of competitive, market-led products being sold, such as agricultural produce and clothing. Disabled youth can participate in income generating projects. This has an effect on their family and friends, as well as the wider community. There are of course still many issues to be addressed in Sierra Leone, including those of poverty and unemployment. The number of children not attending school in Sierra Leone is still estimated to be around 450,000.[33] For those who do attend school, the size

---

[33] Personal communication, UNICEF Sierra Leone May 2006.

of classes – in some cases over 70 pupils – and teacher training and retention are not just disability-related issues, but affect all children in communities. Within economic empowerment programmes, diversity in skills training must be ensured otherwise markets become untenable.

The situation in Sierra Leone exemplifies many of the problems facing disabled people in the longer term recovery and reconstruction of countries affected by conflict, though many of the problems facing disabled people, such as availability of food and water, jobs, education, as well as transport and infrastructure, are the same for the whole community. However, the creation of the DPOs, and the initiation of community based projects such as that in Kabala also demonstrate the potential resources and capabilities that disabled people have. Recovering from the conflict may take years, and necessitates everybody having a role to play. Promoting inclusive education, skills training, micro-credit loans and empowering disabled people to participate in community regeneration not only benefits the local area but also has positive implications for the whole country in terms of reconciliation and peace building.

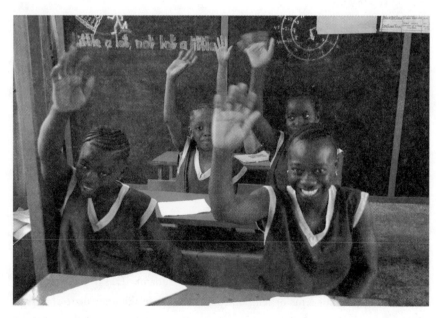

Photo: Jenny Matthews / Leonard Cheshire

The next example from Sri Lanka will focus on the impact of the tsunami on a country affected by years of conflict. The situation demonstrates the complexity of instigating recovery programmes and how disabled people have (however unintentionally) consistently been excluded from many of the reconstruction and rehabilitation programmes.

6. DISABILITY & DISASTERS CASE STUDY: SRI LANKA

There was hardly any warning before the Indian Ocean Tsunami hit the Sri Lankan coastline on 26th December 2004. Roads, hospitals, clinics, houses and whole communities were totally destroyed. The final death toll may never be fully known, but it is estimated over 37,000 people died, and over one million people were made homeless in Sri Lanka alone. A massive international relief effort was implemented, and a huge amount of money was donated to the region. As a result of the tsunami, the World Bank estimated that there was a 20 per cent increase in the number of disabled people in the Asia Pacific region. However, very little money was allocated specifically for disabled people as part of the recovery and reconstruction efforts (Kett et al. 2005).

The situation in Sri Lanka prior to the tsunami was already insecure and uncertain for a number of marginalised groups and individuals. The long running civil war between the government and the Liberation Tigers of the Tamil Eelam (LTTE) is considered the major cause of poverty in Sri Lanka, despite a tentative peace agreement brokered by the Norwegian government in 2001.[34] The conflict has resulted in huge numbers of internally displaced people (IDPs), mainly concentrated in the north and east of the island.[35] These people are inevitably among the poorest sections of the population, often living on less than US$1 per day, and have limited access to employment, housing and education.[36]

As a result of the ongoing conflict in the north and east of the country, an estimated 58 per cent of damaged housing stock remains uninhabitable, almost half of which is in the Batticaloa (east) and Jaffna (north) districts – areas that were badly damaged by the tsunami.[37] By way of example, prior to the tsunami, IDPs in these areas had been waiting years for tents or temporary shelters, yet in the immediate aftermath of the tsunami, over 24,000 were donated, despite only 8,000 tents being required. It is perhaps little wonder that many agencies have been critical of the government's attempts to provide assistance to returnees.[38]

Despite initial collaborative relief efforts, frictions between the government and LTTE re-emerged. Some of these tensions were initially about ongoing needs of tsunami-affected people in conflict-affected areas. This has resulted in a number of agencies (in particular UNHCR) advocating that organisations should focus relief and development efforts on both tsunami and conflict-affected IDPs.[39] These ongoing tensions erupted in February 2005, when E. Kaushalyan (political head of the LTTE in the eastern Batticaloa-Amparai region) was murdered in an ambush in a government-controlled area returning from discussions on post-tsunami relief and recovery work. Five members of his convoy were also killed.[40] Then in early August, Foreign Minister Lakshman Kadirgamar was assassinated at his home in Colombo.

Even prior to the tsunami the identification and registration of people with disabilities was, and is, overall, sporadic and uncoordinated. Therefore it was difficult to gain an accurate picture of the situation in the aftermath, in part as there is a huge variation on how people identify themselves (or are identified by others) as 'disabled', and because of the physical limitations of accounting for all survivors. However, whilst for monitoring and evaluation purposes these may be a prerequisite, merely recording the presence of a disabled person does not mean that they have been included in a programme or project. For example, in Trincomalee, on the east coast, efforts were being made by the Ministry for Social Welfare to compile a database of those with tsunami-related impairments, and their requirements. In practice this only meant equipment and mobility aids etc, and was hampered by a lack of staff and equipment and more 'essential' relief efforts. Inaccurate data and

[34] Department for International Development (DFID).
URL: http://www.dfid.gov.uk/countries/asia/srilanka.asp

[35] There are still more than 350,000 IDPs in Sri Lanka, and non-Tamils displaced from rebel-held areas and Tamils displaced from government high security zones (HSZs), mainly in the north, have been identified as particularly vulnerable to security risks.

[36] http://www.dfid.gov.uk/countries/asia/srilanka.asp

[37] As of October 2004. The Global IDP Project. URL: http://www.db.idpproject.org/Sites/IdpProjectDb/ idpSurvey.nsf/wViewSingleEnv/Sri+LankaProfile+Summary

[38] A UNHCR survey conducted in 2002 demonstrated that over 92 per cent of IDP families needed some form of assistance in order to restart their lives (Global IDP Project)

[39] http://www.db.idpproject.org/Sites/IdpProjectDb/idpSurvey.nsf/wViewSingleEnv/ Sri+LankaProfile+Summary.

[40] Although the actual identities of the killers are not yet known, it is widely believed that they were carried out by forces loyal to Colonel Karuna, who broke away from the LTTE last year. Sri Lanka: Killings Highlight Weaknesses in Ceasefire – Continued Political Violence Threatens Tsunami Relief. URL: http://hrw. org/english/docs/2005/02/11/slanka10162.htm

statistics can have an adverse effect – backing up perceptions that there are 'not that many' disabled people, therefore they do not warrant specific inclusion. Moreover, even if agencies were including disabled people in emergency relief programmes (or at least had guidelines to promote inclusion), there was little evidence that disabled people were being included in longer-term planning, preparedness or mitigation (Kett et al. 2005).

At first glance, Sri Lankan disability legislation seeks to promote equality and inclusion; however, as is common in many countries, there are substantial gaps in its implementation, especially between urban and rural areas, and between conflict- and non-conflict-affected areas. This is perhaps a direct result of two decades of conflict, which particularly affected the north and east of the country. The Disability Organisations Joint Front (DOJF) is the umbrella organisation for disabled people in Sri Lanka. It focuses its attention on common problems such as education, employment, accessibility and legislation. Despite the huge amount of funding available in the aftermath of the tsunami, very little money went to organisations such as the DOJF. However, they worked on gathering information on numbers of disabled people affected by the tsunami; facilitating access to aids and equipment lost during the tsunami; compiling reports on human rights abuses of disabled persons in relief efforts – in particular the stories of disabled people being turned away from temporary camps and shelters, or being unable to access communal water and toilet facilities; as well as participating in the 'Access For All' campaign. This is a network set up by a UK-based NGO specifically in response to the tsunami.[41] Its aim is to push for the accessible reconstruction of all public buildings, transport, places of employment, services and infrastructure, and the inclusion of disabled people in plans for rebuilding the nation.[42]

There are numerous local and INGOs in Sri Lanka committed to protecting the basic rights and the livelihoods of those seen as 'the most vulnerable' in society. NGOs need to work with disabled people and their organisations to ensure that what they are working toward coalesces with the needs of the disabled, and that inclusion is not merely rhetorical. One of the outcomes of the research into inclusion of disabled people in post-conflict and post-disaster relief programmes was the need for DPOs to make links with other civil society organisations to ensure that the voices of

---

[41] http://www.motivation.org.uk/

[42] www.accessforall.lk

disabled people are heard by governments, ministries and other forums. It is also essential that DPOs are recognised as partners in the implementation of relief and development programmes (Kett et al. 2005).

Many local and international organisations shifted their priorities in the immediate aftermath of the tsunami: those already in the field provided immediate aid and relief and in the following days and weeks many other organisations joined in the efforts. This raised the question of who would fill the vacuum left behind in areas less affected by the tsunami?

6.1 MENTAL HEALTH & PSYCHOSOCIAL PROGRAMMES

It was in the area of mental health that this potential vacuum became most obvious. The mental health sector in Sri Lanka is vastly under-resourced – particularly in the north and east, where there is an increase in anxiety, depression, and suicide and, overall, mental health services are short staffed and lack resources (Ashraf 2005). There is apparently very little psychosocial support for people affected by landmines or other explosive remnants of war (ERW), despite a desperate need for this aspect of rehabilitation alongside vocational training and reintegration schemes (Landmine Action 2003). One of the overwhelming responses to the tsunami was the number of psychosocial projects introduced into Sri Lanka.

The issue of post-tsunami trauma counselling and psychosocial care was prominent in many agencies' programmes; for example, in Ampara District on the east coast, at one psychosocial meeting, over 60 NGOs turned up. However, there is something of a dilemma regarding psychosocial programmes, as mental health issues are so stigmatised in Sri Lanka culture, some health professionals differentiate between psychosocial programmes and mental health. The aftermath of the tsunami raised many issues, and although the need for psychosocial care for tsunami 'victims' was deemed essential early on in the recovery process, as one psychiatrist asked, how exactly is a 'tsunami victim' defined? As someone who had lost their family, their home, their job – or is everyone in the society affected in some way? There were also outcomes that had not previously been considered, for example, as many women could not swim to escape the tsunami, there is a large group of single parent fathers who have no previous experience of bringing up children alone and who may well face cultural and family difficulties in trying to adjust and cope with managing a family.

Some healthcare workers and ministers saw this influx of psychosocial projects as beneficial as it would support the fledgling psychiatric service which manifestly would not have been able to cope with the additional strain that was expected after the tsunami. Others felt it did not accurately reflect the scale of the problem, and that a focus on the tsunami may be to the detriment of other services. While the focus on the tsunami may be to the detriment of other services, there was an opportunity for better planning to make mental health programmes, and rehabilitation and reintegration of former patients back into communities, a sustainable and viable option. One of the biggest challenges was to prevent the relapse of people with already existing mental health problems, as these people had already been over-looked prior to the tsunami, and were at risk of being forgotten in the reconstruction phase too.

6.2 CONFLICT, DISASTER & DISABILITY

As this paper has demonstrated, there is often a difference between how those impaired as a result of a disaster or conflict and the 'ordinary' disabled people are treated in both legislation and programming. This difference can manifest in access to both immediate essential requirements and care, as well as in longer-term recovery plans. It may affect issues of compensation – for example, some disabled people we spoke to in Sri Lanka were not injured as a result of the tsunami, nor as a direct result of combat, but as a result of insurgent activities, but were non-combatants (See Box 2). Similar to the group in Sierra Leone, they too had experienced problems with compensation and numerous other barriers, and in several cases, their only compensation had come from organisations allegedly linked to the LTTE.

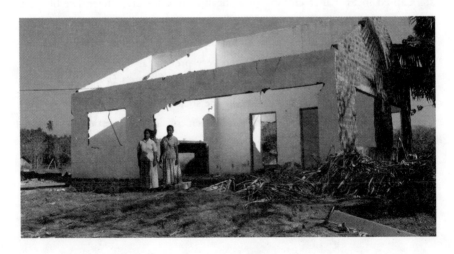

In 2002, a year after the peace negotiations began, Abdul, a 24 year old Tamil man living in Trincomalee, a contested area in the north east of Sri Lanka, was watching a film at a makeshift outdoor cinema in the town with his cousin when terrorists threw a hand grenade into the middle of the audience in an apparently random attack. Several people were killed in the incident, and many more were injured – including Abdul and his cousin. Abdul had severe head and arm injuries, and both he and his cousin lost a leg in the blast. Neither received any government compensation as their injuries were not directly 'conflict-related', and happened after the peace agreement. After a lengthy stay in hospital (only partly paid for by an NGO) Abdul was able to begin rehabilitation. A prosthetic limb was provided through another local NGO and Abdul began to learn to walk again. However, he felt that he could no longer continue his previous college course in computer studies as his family needed him to go to work and earn money, so he took a job selling fish at the local quayside. His livelihood was severely hampered after the tsunami because, as he was not a fisherman, he was not eligible for any of the benefits or relief afforded to tsunami-affected fisherman by the government or NGOs. Even when he did manage to get some fish to sell, people were reluctant to buy them as they were afraid to eat them, fearing them contaminated. The only form of compensation the cousins received came from a rehabilitation organisation linked to the LTTE – as with the situation of IDPs in camps, this raises the question of loyalty and allegiances if money is readily provided.

What the example of Abdul demonstrates is the growing sense of inequality between those affected by the tsunami and those affected by conflict. This manifests from both national legislations and policies, as well as practices in relief and development. The situation remains politically tense in Sri Lanka over a year on from the tsunami. Many people are still living in temporary accommodation and reconstruction is still ongoing. LCI have set up a Disability Resource Centre in Colombo, with two outreach offices in the east of the country. They provide advice and support for disabled people and their families and help find ways to redress some of these inequalities.

7. CONCLUSIONS

Disabled people face numerous barriers to inclusion in society, despite the work of various organisations and legislations. However, this exclusion can have dire consequences in extreme situations of conflict and disasters, as the examples here have demonstrated. The cases outlined here only briefly touch on the barriers disabled people face against being included in relief and development efforts following disasters or conflicts, from access to emergency relief through to the whole issue of national legislation and compensation. There are of course also many responses, which shift according to location, time, gender, age, ethnicity, and a myriad of other factors besides. But despite the (obvious) links, disabled people have been largely ignored in international relief and development efforts in this area. This is partly because it is still a relatively under-researched (and under-funded) area, and much more work needs to be undertaken to fill in some of the gaps. Much of the work is carried out by DPOs who remain outside mainstream development. INGOs therefore need to ensure that they work with DPOs on an equal basis so they can join in wider relief and development debates.

Central to the issue of linking relief and development is addressing poverty. Tackling the question of poverty requires global solutions, and is linked to broader issues such as human security, environmental protection and gender inequalities. Disabled people, their families, and organisations need to establish links with other organisations and civil society movements to ensure that their voices are added to the debates around these issues. Such links strengthen the position of all concerned, and ensure that those who are advocating similar things do so from a similar position.

DPOs and other civil society organisations need to be strengthened prior to a disaster or emergency happening, so they have adequate resources to respond quickly to the needs of disabled people and work with INGOs and donors. As the examples from Sierra Leone and Sri Lanka demonstrate, disabled people and DPOs need to be involved from early on to ensure meaningful consultation and collaboration. They have already existing networks and can be involved in raising awareness about mainstreaming disability into all aspects of emergency planning, response and reconstruction efforts. Building on these opportunities may necessitate capacity building, as well as fundamental shifts in attitudes and beliefs. Local communities and DPOs can provide specific advice and expertise to the different stages of disaster mitigation, responses, and recovery planning, especially training.

The process of recovering from a disaster or conflict is both individual and social. Governments in disaster or conflict-affected countries need to have available the resources needed for inclusive community development. But recovery may also require facilities for psychosocial rehabilitation, CBR projects, education pro- grammes for families and communities, and microfinance initiatives to help promote integration and rehabilitation. Including disabled people in community- based programmes can have positive implications for post-conflict and post-disaster reconstruction and development, provided they do not become the 'gold standard' to get people to be economically productive. Inclusion and community participation improves individual decision-making capacity, self-esteem, and confidence, which in turn can have a positive impact on a community. This in turn may contribute to the promotion of security, reconciliation and reintegration in disaster and conflict-affected countries. For many disabled people, barriers to participation within communities are primarily social and cultural, rather than a direct result of impairments. Programmes which focus on meaningful participation and inclusion of disabled people who can offer practical explanations of what still needs to be done with and by disabled people, using local knowledge and resources offer a much higher chance of success in communities affected by disasters and conflict.

REFERENCES

Ashraf, A., 2005. Tsunami wreaks mental health havoc. *Bulletin of the World Health Organisation* [online], 83 (6). Available from: http://www.who.int/bulletin/ volumes/83/6/infocus0605/en/index1.html

Baingana, F., and Bannon, I., 2004 *Integrating Mental Health and Psychosocial Interventions into World Bank Lending for Conflict-Affected Populations: A Toolkit.* World Bank Conflict Prevention and Reconstruction Unit. Available from: http://lnweb18.worldbank.org/ESSD/sdvext.nsf/67ByDocName/ IntegratingMentalHealthandPsychosocialinterventionsintoWorldBankLend- ConflictAffectedPopulationAToolkit/$FILE/Tookkit-Final.pdf

Banatvala, N., and Zwi, A., 2000. Public health and humanitarian interventions: developing the evidence base. *British Medical Journal* 321: 101-105.

Boyce, W., 2000. Disability Problems and Rehabilitation Responses in an Era of Armed Conflict. *Disability and the Third World* 11 (3): 88-96.

Boyce, W., Koros, M., and Hodgson, J., 2002. Community based rehabilitation: a strategy for peace-building. *BMC International Health and Human Rights* [online] (2) 6. Available from: http://www.biomedcentral.com/content/pdf/1472-698X-2-6.pdf

Coleridge, P., 1998. Development, Cultural Values and Disability: The Example of Afghanistan. *Conference on Disability Issues: Global Solutions and the Role of Community Based Rehabilitation,* Queen's University, Kingston, Canada: March 5-6. Available from: http://www.eenet.org.uk/key_issues/cultural/colerdge1.shtml

Commission on Human Security, 2003. *Human Security Now.* New York: CHS Available from: http://www.humansecuritychs.org/finalreport/English/FinalReport.pdf

Edmonds, L.J., 2005. Mainstreaming community based rehabilitation in primary health care in Bosnia-Herzegovina. *Disability & Society* 20 (3): 293-309.

Finkenflügel, H., 2006. Who is in… And what for? An analysis of stakeholders' influences in CBR. *Asia Pacific Disability Rehabilitation Journal* 17 (1).

Giacaman, R., 2001. A community of citizens: disability rehabilitation in the Palestinian transition to statehood. *Disability and Rehabilitation* 23 (14): 639-644.

Harris, A. & Enfield, S., 2003. *Disability, Equality, and Human Rights: A Training Manual for Development and Humanitarian Organisations.* Oxford: Oxfam GB (in association with Action on Disability and Development).

Hoogeveen, JG., 2005. Measuring Welfare for Small but Vulnerable Groups: Poverty and Disability in Uganda. *Journal of African Economies* 14 (4): 603-631.

IDDC, 2000. Disability and Conflict Report of IDDC Seminar May 29th – June 4th. [online] Available from: http://www.iddc.org.uk/dis_dev/key_issues/dis_confl_rep.doc

IDDC, 2004. Inclusive Development and the UN Convention: IDDC Reflection Paper [online] Available from: http://www.un.org/esa/socdev/enable/rights/ahc3iddc.pdf

ILO, UNESCO and WHO, 2004. *CBR: A Strategy for the rehabilitation, equalization of opportunities, Poverty Reduction and Social Inclusion of People with Disabilities. Joint position paper 2004.* Switzerland: WHO.

Inclusion International, 2005. *Fact sheet on poverty and disability* [online] London: Inclusion International. Available from: http://www.inclusioninternational.org/ site_uploads/11223821811255866183.pdf

Jones, R.A., 2006. No alternative: post-war poverty reduction as structural transformation in Rwanda. *Conflict, Security & Development* 6 (2) 151-178.

Kett, M. and Mannion, S., 2004. Managing the Health Effects of the Explosive Remnants of War. *Journal of the Royal Society for the Promotion of Health* 124/6.

Kett, M., Stubbs, S., and Yeo, R., 2005. Disability in Conflict and Emergency Situations. International Disability and Development Consortium. Report for DFiD Disability Knowledge and Research Programme [online] available from: http://www.disabilitykar.net/docs/thematic_conflict.doc

Landmine Action, 2003. ERW in Sri Lanka. London: Landmine Action. Available from: http://www.landmineaction.org/resources/ERW_Sri_Lanka.pdf

Médecins Sans Frontières, 1997. *Refugee Health.* London: McMillan.

Murray, C., King, G., Lopez, A., Tomijima, N., and Krug, E., 2002. Armed conflict as a public health problem. *BMJ* 324:346-349.

National Organization on Disability [no date] *Report on Special Needs Assessment for Katrina Evacuees (SNAKE) project.* Washington DC: NOD. Available from: http://www.nod.org/Resources/PDFs/katrina_snake_report.pdf

van Ommeren, M., Saxena, S., & Saraceno, B., 2005. Mental and social health during and after acute emergencies: emerging consensus? *Bulletin of the World Health Organization* 83 (1).

Parr, A.R., 1987. Disasters and disabled persons; An examination of the safety needs of a neglected minority. *Disasters* (11) 2.

SHIA / WHO, 2002. *Community Based Rehabilitation As We Have Experienced It... Voices of Persons With Disabilities.* Geneva: World Health Organisation. Available from: http://whqlibdoc.who.int/publications/9241590432.pdf

Slaymaker, T., Christiansen, K., with Hemming, I., 2005. *Community-based approaches and service delivery: Issues and options in difficult environments and partnerships.* Overseas Development Institute. Available from: http://www.id21. org/zinter/id21zinter.exe?a=i&w=s10cts1g1

Sphere Project, 2004. *Sphere Humanitarian Charter and Minimum Standards in Disaster Response* (4th edition) Geneva: Sphere Project. Available from: http://www.sphereproject.org/handbook/index.htm

UNHCR, 1995. Post-Conflict Recovery: UNHCRs Capacities and Perspectives. International Colloquium on Post-Conflict Reconstruction Strategies: 1-16. Available from: http://66.102.9.104/search?q=cache:ZjFro-3nZq0J:www.metafro. be/grandslacs/grandslacsdir300/2413.pdf+post+conflict+recovery:+unhcr%27s+ca pacities+and+perspectives&hl=en

United Nations Development Programme, 1994. *Human Development Report.* New York and Oxford: Oxford University Press. Available from: http://hdr.undp.org/reports/global/1994/en/

United Nations High Commissioner for Refugees, 1996. *Assisting disabled refugees: a community-based approach.* (2nd ed) Geneva: UNHCR.

World Health Organisation, 2002. *World Report on Violence and Health.* Geneva: WHO. Available from: http://www.who.int/violence_injury_prevention/violence/ world_report/en/full_en.pdf

WHO, 2006. Disability and Rehabilitation WHO Action Plan 2006-2011. Geneva: WHO. Available from: http://www.who.int/disabilities/publications/dar_ action_plan_2006to2011.pdf

WHO, 2001. *World Health Report 2001: Mental health: new understanding, new hope.* Geneva: WHO.

World Bank, 2005a. Examining Inclusion: Disability and Community Driven Development. Social Development Notes 100. Washington: World Bank. Available from: http://siteresources.worldbank.org/DISABILITY/Resources/ Community-Based-Rehabilitation/Examining_Inclusion.pdf

World Bank, 2005b. *Overview of Disabled Persons Organizations (DPOs) Working in Tsunami-Affected Areas* [online] Available from: http://web.worldbank.org/WBSITE/EXTERNAL/TOPICS/EXTSOCIAL PROTECTION/EXTDISABILITY/0,,contentMDK:20319525~pagePK: 148956~piPK:216618~theSitePK :282699,00.html#Asia_and_Pacific_ Development_Center_on_Disability_APCD